Animal Production and Health: Safety and Risk Management

Animal Production and Health: Safety and Risk Management

Aaron Dixon

Larsen & Keller
www.larsen-keller.com

Animal Production and Health: Safety and Risk Management
Aaron Dixon
ISBN: 979-8-88836-049-1 (Hardback)

Larsen & Keller
Published by Larsen and Keller Education,
5 Penn Plaza,
19th Floor,
New York, NY 10001, USA

Cataloging-in-Publication Data

Animal production and health : safety and risk management / Aaron Dixon.
p. cm.
Includes bibliographical references and index.
ISBN 979-8-88836-049-1
1. Animal culture. 3. Animal health. 3. Livestock. 4. Animal industry--Safety measures.
I. Dixon, Aaron.
SF615 .A55 2023
636.089--dc23

For more information regarding Larsen and Keller Education and its products, please visit the publisher's website www.larsen-keller.com

Table of Contents

Preface

Animal science studies the biology, health, production and management of animals, which are of economic interest to humans. It integrates the studies of genetics, animal physiology, reproduction and microbiology. Animal production involves raising animals for the purpose of obtaining meat, fiber, milk or any other product. Animal health is studied within the discipline of veterinary medicine. It involves the management, treatment and prevention of animal diseases and injuries. Animal health is also a significant aspect of public health, since a number of diseases, known as zoonoses, can be transferred from animals to humans. Research in animal production and veterinary medicine transcends species boundaries and also works at human-animal interfaces such as food safety and ecosystem health. This book is compiled in such a manner, that it will provide in-depth knowledge about safety and risk management with respect to animal production and health. For all readers who are interested in these topics, the studies included herein will serve as an excellent guide to develop a comprehensive understanding.

The researches compiled throughout the book are authentic and of high quality, combining several disciplines and from very diverse regions from around the world. Drawing on the contributions of many researchers from diverse countries, the book's objective is to provide the readers with the latest achievements in the area of research. This book will surely be a source of knowledge to all interested and researching the field.

In the end, I would like to express my deep sense of gratitude to all the authors for meeting the set deadlines in completing and submitting their research chapters. I would also like to thank the publisher for the support offered to us throughout the course of the book. Finally, I extend my sincere thanks to my family for being a constant source of inspiration and encouragement.

Aaron Dixon

1

Veterinary Services: Roles and Responsibilities

Gary Vroegindewey

National Veterinary Services have a wide range of regulatory and operational responsibilities as directed by their respective countries. These responsibilities could include animal health, animal welfare, food safety, zoonotic disease surveillance and control, import and export regulations, trade in livestock and livestock products, disaster management, and other functional areas (OIE 2017). In many cases veterinary services are resourced to meet minimal capability needed for animal health and trade. Therefore, veterinary services may lack the authorities and capacities to meet the unique requirements presented in disaster situations including NREs.

Disasters by definition are those events that exceed the normal capacity to respond at some level (Akshat 2017). Animals and animal-related issues are increasingly part of disaster management and risk reduction due to their economic, health, welfare, and social aspects (PETS ACT 2006). In addition to the livestock and food chain issues, National Veterinary Services may be called on to prepared for and respond to NREs in other special animal categories such as search and rescue animals, service animals, laboratory animals, zoo and aquatic exhibition animals, and wildlife.

Veterinary services are generally trained and experienced in dealing with biological animal disasters such at the incursion of a transboundary disease of economic importance to the livestock industry such as African swine fever or foot-and-mouth disease. However, there is less experience and capability to deal with non-biological disasters such as floods, drought, earthquakes, tornadoes, volcanic eruption, and extreme weather events. The foundation for National Veterinary Services in general, and disaster preparedness and response specifically is the legislative framework and authorities to perform specified functions. National legislation

G. Vroegindewey (✉)
College of Veterinary Medicine, Lincoln Memorial University, Harrogate, TN, USA
e-mail: Gary.Vroegindewey@lmunet.edu

needs to be reviewed to ensure veterinary service disaster management and disaster risk reduction authorities are included. National disaster preparedness and contingency plans should address the animal health and welfare component and detail the roles and responsibilities of each department and ministry including the lead authority for each type of event. National Veterinary Services should use these documents to develop an all-hazards approach for their specific disaster preparedness contingency plans (AVMA 2012). Technological disasters such as chemical spills, toxic gas releases, and NREs present an even greater challenge since many veterinary services will not have authorities and capabilities established for these types of events (Vroegindewey 2014).

Global natural and climate disasters in 2017 affected over 95 million people with over 9600 deaths, costing over $335 billion dollars (US) (CRED 2017). Many if not most of these disasters have an animal component that requires veterinary response. The need for effective local, national, regional, and international capabilities is highlighted by the United Nations Office for Disaster Risk Reduction (UNISDR) Sendai Framework for Disaster Risk Reduction 2015–2030 (UNISDR 2015) that builds on the previous Hyogo Framework for Action 2005–2015 Building the Resilience of Nations and Communities to Disasters (UNISDR 2005). These two documents provide a framework for nations to build their own disaster preparedness, disaster contingency, and disaster risk reduction plans. Included in the Sendai framework are seven global targets:

(i) To reduce mortality
(ii) Reduce impacted individuals
(iii) Reduce economic loss
(iv) Reduce infrastructure damage and disruption of basics services
(v) Increase national risk reduction strategies
(vi) Enhance international cooperation
(vii) Increase the availability and access to multi-hazard early warning systems and disaster risk information and assessments

In addition, there are four priorities for action including understanding disaster risk, strengthening disaster risk governance, investing in disaster risk reduction, and enhancing disaster preparedness. These targets and priorities for action can be used by intergovernmental organizations, governments, and National Veterinary Services as a roadmap toward building efficient and effective disaster management programs including those addressing NREs.

A study conducted by the World Organization for Animal Health (OIE) in 2014 on the preparedness of National Veterinary Services to respond to natural disasters and bioterrorism demonstrated significant gaps in authorities and capabilities (Vroegindewey 2014). The study surveyed European and Western Asian countries' National Veterinary Services with 48 responses out of 53 countries queried. There was a wide range of responses on national legislation and incorporation of animal-focused disaster management into National Disaster Response Plans. Twenty-one percent of the respondents indicated that no national legislation addressed animals in disasters. Sixty-six percent of the countries indicated the absence of guidelines, standards, handbooks, and references for dealing with disasters. While livestock was covered by 81% of the National Disaster Response Plans, there were fewer plans that covered companion animals (52%), zoo and aquatic exhibit animals (52%), and wildlife (42%). A review of the OIE list of Performance of Veterinary Services publicly published evaluations indicated only 4 of 27 National Veterinary Services had the highest level of residue surveillance programs including radionuclides and 17 of 27 had no or very limited capacity reported (OIE 2019). These numbers underscore the scope of work that veterinary services will need to accomplish to meet the needs of society in disaster scenarios including NREs. Many National Veterinary Services did not use guidelines for disaster preparedness and response despite the availability of numerous international publications and guidelines for National Veterinary Services to meet these disaster-focused operational requirements.

OIE has published general guidelines such as OIE Guidelines on Disaster Management and Risk Reduction in Relation to Animal Health and Welfare and Veterinary Public Health (OIE 2016). This guideline provides general principles for disaster management. The OIE Terrestrial Animal Health Code 2017 (OIE 2017) provides high-level guidance on legislative authorities and operational guidelines for animal disease incursions but limited information on disasters with the primary focus on mass depopulation and disposal of animals in natural disaster and disease situations. There are no specific references for NREs included. The United Nation Food and Agricultural Organization (FAO) has published the Good Emergency Management Practice: The Essentials, a comprehensive guide for preparing for and responding to animal health emergencies (FAO 2011). This detailed guide focuses on animal health emergencies with an emphasis on Transboundary Animal Diseases (TAD). It can be used as a framework to develop veterinary service preparedness plans, contingency plans, operational plans, and standard operating procedures (SOP), which can be used to easily integrate the requirements of the existing IAEA standards on preparedness and response to NREs.

One area that has not been significantly addressed in standards and guidelines is the need for training in behavioral health resilience and providing medical and behavioral health support to responders before, during, and after the termination of the emergency phases of a disaster event.

Disaster risk management (DRM) has emerged as a focus in the international disaster management for identifying risk and risk analysis to prepare for, mitigate, and respond to disasters. FAO published a guideline disaster risk management systems analysis (FAO 2008) that details the process for DRM and provides a toolbox for development of protection strategies in line with IAEA requirements.

NREs such as Chernobyl, Fukushima Daiichi, Kyshtym, Windscale, and Three Mile Island illustrate the potential for radiological events that would require national veterinary service preparedness and response. The IAEA has published numerous requirements and guidelines that are relevant to the National Veterinary Services for NREs. The IAEA publication Joint Radiation Emergency Management Plan of the International Organizations provides (IAEA 2013) high-level national and regional guidance for management of NRE with specific functions and organizational links for information and support (IAEA 2002a). Food and food chain issues are addressed in this document.

The IAEA safety standards detail general requirements and specific guidelines which are applicable to veterinary service responders. IAEA safety standard Preparedness and Response for a Nuclear or Radiological Emergency GSR-7, 2015, outlines the general high-level requirements for preparing for and responding to NREs (IAEA 2015). This set of requirements include:

- A framework for emergency preparedness and response
- The lessons learned from past emergencies
- An internally consistent foundation for the application of principles of and insights into radiation protection
- A framework for developing an explanation of the criteria for the public and for public officials to address the risks of radiation exposure to human health and for a proportionate response

The IAEA General Safety Guide GSG-2, 2011, Criteria for Use in Preparedness and Response for a Nuclear or Radiological Emergency (IAEA 2011) provides a starting point for veterinary services to train personnel. The safety guide was cosponsored by FAO, the World Health Organization (WHO), the Pan American Health Organization (PAHO), and the International Labour Office (ILO). The overall goal of GSG-2 is to "Present a coherent set of generic criteria that form a basis for developing the operational levels needed for decision making concerning protective actions and other response actions necessary to meet the emergency response objectives."

In addition to the criteria, Operational Interventional Level (OIL) provides guidance for responders to take appropriate actions. The IAEA defines the OILs (IAEA 2017) as "A calculated level, measured by instruments in the field or determined by laboratory analysis, that corresponds to an intervention level or action level. OILs are typically expressed in terms of dose rates or of activity of radioactive material released, time integrated air concentration, ground or surface concentration or activity concentrations of radionuclides in environmental food or water samples. An OIL is a type of action level that is used immediately and directly (without further assessment) to determine the appropriate protective actions on the basis of an environmental measurement."

OIL values for food, milk, and drinking water and associated actions provide a baseline for veterinary service decision-making in NREs (IAEA 2017). For example, at OIL 3 the criteria state:

> If other food is available in the territories where OIL 3 is exceeded, stop consuming local produce (e.g., vegetables), milk from grazing animals and rainwater until they have been screened and declared safe. However, if restriction of consumption is likely to result in severe malnutrition or dehydration because replacement food, milk or water is not available, these items may be consumed for a short time until replacements are available.

These plain language criteria based on technical data provide National Veterinary Services with a defensible basis that can be used to explain the rationale for actions to be taken during a NRE.

The IAEA General Safety Guide GSG-11, 2018, Arrangements for the Termination of a Nuclear or Radiological Emergency (IAEA 2018b) provides guidelines that can be used by veterinary services to support operational response activities to assist in termination of the NRE. The document specifies that food, milk, and drinking water restrictions may continue after the termination of the NRE due to the continued risk to public health from products in the food chain and continued contamination to livestock, water, and foodstuffs. Monitoring will be required to ensure that agricultural products meet international trade standards. Comprehensive routine monitoring programs would be established until acceptable levels are achieved.

Codex Alimentarius has published the CODEX General Standard for Contaminants and Toxins in Food and Feed (CODEX STAN 193–1995) (CODEX 2015) that "lists the maximum levels and associated sampling plans of contaminants and natural toxicants in food and feed which are recommended by the CAC to be applied to commodities moving in international trade." It also states that "This standard includes only maximum levels of contaminants and natural toxicants in feed in cases where the contaminant in feed can be transferred to food of animal origin and can be relevant for public health." These guidelines are established for radionuclides in foods that are traded internationally for human consumption; however, the criteria can be applied in conjunction with a national standard which may be more restrictive (FAO-WHO 1989).

Guidelines and standards are critical to but not sufficient for effective NRE preparedness and response. National Veterinary Services need to integrate the requirements and recommendations of these standards. These requirements can be broken down into several organizational and operational components: legislation, leadership, organization, training, personnel, material, facilities, and finance.

Specific veterinary service contingency plans and standard operating procedures (SOP) for NREs should be developed and coordinated across government departments and ministries and be reflected in the regional and national plans.

Veterinary leadership at the national, departmental, and ministry level must be committed to the preparation for, and response to NREs. Effective preparedness and response plan would include the following:

- Conducting NRE risk analysis
- Understanding the unique aspects of NRE events
- Understanding the role of the veterinary service in the context of national disaster management plans
- Creating veterinary service contingency and operational plans
- Building, training, and exercising a NRE-capable workforce
- Acquiring required materials and facilities
- Creating an appropriate organizational structure
- Securing resources to accomplish these tasks

National Veterinary Services need to develop the organizational capacity to prepare for and respond to NREs. This includes developing the structures and personnel to work at the field level, veterinary headquarter levels, and national emergency operations/coordination center. Trained designated personnel should be available to direct the veterinary response, communicate with national and regional authorities, and communicate with the public and animal health stakeholders as well as intergovernmental organizations (IGO) such as IAEA, OIE, FAO, WHO, and other IGO entities. Stakeholders are any individual or group that has an interest in any decision or activity of an organization (ISO 2010). Specific units need to be identified as the lead for each of the functions required for preparedness and response. Veterinary service personnel need to be identified and trained to fill each contingency and operational plan role from field work to headquarters to national operation centers. Laboratory personnel need to be trained and available to accomplish required analysis that may be outside the normal scope of day-to-day testing.

Training and education are key components for National Veterinary Services personnel. While generally experienced in dealing with day-to-day animal health and welfare issues, many are not trained and experienced in dealing with technological disasters such as NREs. The OIE recommendation guideline Competency of Graduate Veterinarians ("Day 1 graduates") to assure National Veterinary Services of Quality (OIE 2012) includes risk analysis as a competency but does not include competency in disaster management and disaster risk reduction nor specific competencies in NRE capabilities. Therefore, new graduates and veterinary personnel will need to be trained, educated, and assessed on their skills in this arena. The training should include all personnel with a designated task in NREs. This includes leadership, headquarters, field operations, laboratory, and other functional areas. The training can include technical training such as performing specific laboratory analysis for radionuclides in animal or food samples; use of dosimeters and monitoring devices; proper use of personal protective equipment (PPE); decontamination, destruction, and disposal of contaminated food and nonfood materials; as well as nontechnical operational requirements. Examples of these nontechnical skills are risk assessment, risk communications, team building, working in national emergency operation centers, developing NRE contingency plans and SOP, and similar operational and organizational skillsets. Training is accomplished at the individual level, team level, and the organizational level. Training should be tracked by individual and organization to ensure there is complete coverage, newly hired personnel are trained, and refresher training and recertification are accomplished. The effectiveness of the training should be validated through testing and exercising the response plans and modified to meet any training gaps that are identified.

Veterinary personnel will need to be hired, trained, and assessed through all levels of the organization for both day-to-day operations and emergency operations such as a NRE event. Backup and reserve personnel need to be identified for each function position. Critical positions should be identified and resourced. Prior experiences with NRE events such as the Japan Earthquake-Tsunami-Fukushima reactor NRE demonstrate that veterinary service personnel in the affected area may be part of the affected population and unable to effectively perform their assigned duties;

therefore a backup system of trained personnel should be available (OIE 2019). Increased workload during a NRE event may require adding personnel to cover the expanded scope of the event, and these added personnel will also require refresher or just-in-time training and equipping. Additional personnel required can be established through bilateral and regional mutual support agreements, establishing and training a reserve veterinary force, coordinating with the military as part of Military Support to Civilian Operations, and contracting civilian personnel.

National Veterinary Services will need to identify and acquire the material needed to train for and respond to NREs. Some of these materials are not used daily and may require special purchasing, stockpiling, and maintaining with a logistical distribution plan. The specific types of items that may be required for a NRE include personal dosimeters, various types of in situ radiation monitoring devices, PPE, specialized radiation detection laboratory equipment, decontamination facilities, and other items. General emergency response materials will be required including communications equipment, computers, transportation assets, protective sheltering, animal handling equipment, and other general use items.

National Veterinary Services will need to identify and acquire facilities sufficient to conduct daily operations as well as contingency operations at the national, regional, and local level. Increased space may be required to meet the operational surge of response activity and may be pre-identified and contracted for before an event. Emergency operation centers, increased laboratory requirements, decontamination areas, and animal carcass disposal sites must be considered. Contingency plans should identify critical infrastructure requirements and where those activities would take place in case that facility is within an exclusion zone.

Resourcing for National Veterinary Services to execute daily and emergent operations can be a challenge. Requirements for material, personnel, facilities, and operational activities should be identified and brought to the national governmental level for legislative and funding support. Funding should be identified for compensation for livestock that may need to be depopulated. Even if this level of funding is unlikely to be committed ahead of a disaster having a NRE, the existence of operational requirements document will expedite the release of funds.

National Veterinary Services have multiple resources beyond these guidelines to meet their operational requirements for NREs. OIE has expanded its disaster focus beyond animal diseases to include all hazards and is incorporating disaster training into its operational mandate (OIE 2016). The WHO, OIE, and FAO have collaborated on sharing responsibilities and coordinating global activities to address health risks at the animal-human-ecosystems interfaces. The focus of this Tripartite Concept Note is with animal and zoonotic diseases, but these collaborative relationships can be built upon for other disasters including NREs (FAO-OIE-WHO 2010). The IAEA has launched a program to support National Veterinary Services (IAEA 2018a) to address multiple facets of NRE preparedness and response including:

- Legislative/strategies
- Containment and management of containment
- Detection and differentiation

- Development of guidelines (contingency plan)
- Simulation exercise and sharing information

In addition, the Joint FAO/IAEA Programme of Nuclear Techniques in Food and Agriculture provides a concept of operations for notification and advisory information (IAEA 2019).

In 2005 the IAEA established the Incident and Emergency Centre (IEC – https://www.iaea.org/about/organizational-structure/department-of-nuclear-safety-and-security/incident-and-emergency-centre) which is the global focal point for international emergency preparedness, communication, and response to nuclear and radiological incidents and emergencies, regardless of whether they arise from accident, negligence, or deliberate act. It is the world's center for the coordination of international emergency preparedness and response assistance. This center was created in response to the increase use of nuclear applications as well as emerging issues of the intentional malicious use of nuclear and radiological material. The IEC operates the IAEA Incident and Emergency System (IES). The IEC has four focus areas: IES Preparedness, IES Operation, Member State preparedness, and emergency communications and outreach. These last two focus areas could support National Veterinary Services to prepare for, and respond to NREs.

The IES includes training, emergency response exercising, and on-call capability. The IES activities are in compliance with the Convention on Early Notification of a Nuclear Accident (IAEA 2002b) and the Convention on Assistance in the Case of a Nuclear Accident or Radiological Emergency (IAEA 2002a), including operations of the IAEA Response and Assistance Network (RANET) and the ability to provide assistance mission upon request. They can assist Member States in developing their emergency preparedness and response framework and arrangements and provide safety standards and other technical guidance, education and training, and conducting Emergency Preparedness Reviews (EPREV missions). Specific guidance and advice are available for essential tasks such as public communication for NREs through different IAEA publications on public communication and provision of training on these topics.

National Veterinary Services have critical roles in the preparedness and response to NREs to protect public health through control of products of animal origin. Assessment of current NRE risks, authorities, and capabilities would be a starting point to identify needs to meet governmental and societal responsibilities. The complexity of NREs in regard to National Veterinary Services can be seen in these four major NREs. Using these models of NREs, National Veterinary Services can do an assessment of what roles and responsibilities they would need to fulfill to have an efficient and effective response to meet their designated requirements.

The Kyshtym NRE in the Urals of the USSR was not a nuclear power plant accident; it was a release of radionuclides from a storage tank due to the failure of a cooling system. In the early phase after the NRE, the major contributor to the dose to humans was the internal exposure from ^{144}Ce and ^{95}Zr largely from crops (Standring et al. 2009). The maximum concentration of ^{144}Ce or ^{95}Zr in agricultural products on land closest to source areas (up to 20 km) reached 10–10,000 kBq/kg.

For milk, the key isotope contributing to internal dose was long-lived ^{90}Sr and, to a much lesser extent, ^{137}Cs.

The Windscale NRE occuredwhen there was a buildup of Wigner energy which led to a fire that released radionuclides into the atmosphere in the north of the UK. Milk from dairy cows grazing adjacent lowland areas was contaminated by short-lived ^{131}I, and a limit was set for radioiodine in milk of 0.1 μCi/L (3700 Bq/L). Sheep grazing upland areas were also contaminated by ^{137}Cs. Po-210 may also have contaminated animal tissues but received little attention at the time.

The Chernobyl NRE occurred during an experiment when there was a surge of power followed by two explosions. There was a release of radionuclides over a period of 10 days, and the fallout contaminated large areas of the terrestrial environment with a major impact on both agricultural animal production and extensive animal production on poor land and game animal harvesting largely from forests. The most severely affected areas within 100 km of the nuclear power plant in the USSR were Ukraine, Belarus, and the Russian Federation, but other areas of Eastern and Western Europe were also contaminated, especially where the passage of the contaminated fallout in the atmosphere coincided with heavy rainfall. Therefore, problems with animal products were widely experienced not only within the former Soviet Union but also in many other countries in Europe (USSR Ministry Agriculture 1977).

After the Fukushima Daiichi NRE in Japan there was a system failure that led to a loss of cooling capacity of the power plant and resulted in several releases of radionuclides due to venting and hydrogen explosions. These releases contributed to contamination of agricultural areas. A key difference in this event compared with the other NREs is that animal products were relatively less contaminated because most dairy and other livestock animals are housed indoors in Japan.

Numerous national, regional, and international guidelines and resources are available to support the strengthening of National Veterinary Services to prepare for and respond to all disasters and particularly the unique complex issues present with NREs. Understanding the requirements, planning and preparing, training, and exercising National Veterinary Service capabilities and capacities will better prepare National Veterinary Services to perform their role and responsibilities in NREs. This will support the protection of animal health and welfare and veterinary public health and maintain the economic viability of the animal sector.

References

Akshat, R. (2017). *Global disasters in 2017 cost $306 billion – Nearly double the cost of 2016.* https://qz.com/1162791/2017-natural-disasters-and-climate-change-effects-cost-the-world-306-billion/

AVMA. (2012). *Emergency preparedness and response.* https://ebusiness.avma.org/files/product-downloads/emerg_prep_resp_guide.pdf

CODEX STAN. (2015). *FAO-WHO CODEX General Standard for Contaminants and Toxins in Food and Feed 193–1995.* http://www.fao.org/input/download/standards/17/CXS_193e_2015.pdf

CRED. (2017). Center for Research on the Epidemiology of Disasters (CRED) Natural Disasters 2017.

FAO. (2008). *Disaster risk management systems analysis – A guide book.* ISSN 1684 8241. http://www.fao.org/3/a-i0304e.pdf

FAO. (2011). *FAO good emergency management practice: The essentials – A guide to preparing for animal health emergencies.* ISSN 1810-1119. http://www.fao.org/3/a-ba0137e.pdf

FAO-OIE-WHO. (2010). *The FAO-OIE-WHO Collaboration – Sharing responsibilities and coordinating global activities to address health risks at the animal-human-ecosystems interfaces – A Tripartite Concept Note.* http://www.fao.org/3/ak736e/ak736e00.pdf

FAO-WHO. (1989). *Guideline levels for radionuclides in foods following accidental nuclear contamination for use in international trade.* CAC/GL 5–1989. http://www.criirad.org/actualites/dossiers2005/menacesradioactivesaliments/codexanglais1989.pdf

IAEA. (2002a). *Convention on assistance in the case of a nuclear accident or radiological emergency.* https://www.iaea.org/sites/default/files/publications/documents/infcircs/1986/infcirc335a11-infcirc336a12.pdf

IAEA. (2002b). *Convention on early notification of a nuclear accident.* https://www.iaea.org/sites/default/files/publications/documents/infcircs/1986/infcirc335a11-infcirc336a12.pdf

IAEA. (2011). *IAEA safety standards GSG-2, 2011, criteria for use in preparedness and response for a nuclear or radiological emergency.* https://iaea.org/publications/8506/criteria-for-use-in-preparedness-and-response-for-a nuclear-or-radiologicalemergency

IAEA. (2013). *Joint radiation emergency management plan of the international organizations – EPR–JPLAN.* https://www-pub.iaea.org/MTCD/Publications/PDF/EPRJplan2013_web.pdf

IAEA. (2015). *Preparedness and response for a nuclear or radiological emergency – General safety requirements.* GSR Part 7. https://www-pub.iaea.org/MTCD/Publications/PDF/P_1708_web.pdf

IAEA. (2017). *Operational intervention levels for reactor emergencies and methodology for their derivation.* https://www-pub.iaea.org/MTCD/Publications/PDF/EPR_NPP_OILs_2017_web.pdf

IAEA. (2018a). *IAEA project RER/9/137 – Enhancing national capabilities for response to nuclear and radiological emergencies.* https://iaea.org/projects/tc/rer9137

IAEA. (2018b). *IAEA publication GSG-11, 2018, Arrangements for the termination of a nuclear or radiological emergency.* https://iaea.org/publications/12269/arrangements-for-the-termination-of-a-nuclear-or-radiological-emergency

IAEA. (2019). *Joint FAO/IAEA programme for nuclear for techniques in food and agriculture; preparedness and response to nuclear emergencies.* http://www-naweb.iaea.org/nafa/fep/topic-nuclear-emergencies.html

ISO 26000. (2010). *Guidance on social responsibility.* https://iso.org/iso-26000-social-responsibility.html

OIE. (2012). *OIE recommendations on the Competencies of graduating veterinarians ('Day 1 graduates') to assure National Veterinary Services of quality.* http://www.oie.int/fileadmin/Home/eng/Support_to_OIE_Members/Vet_Edu_AHG/DAY_1/DAYONE-B-ang-vC.pdf

OIE. (2016). *OIE guidelines on disaster management and risk reduction in relation to animal health and welfare and veterinary public health.* http://www.oie.int/fileadmin/Home/eng/Animal_Welfare/docs/pdf/Others/Disastermanagement-ANG.pdf

OIE. (2017). *OIE terrestrial animal health code.* http://www.oie.int/standard-setting/terrestrial-code/access-online/

OIE. (2019). *PVS evaluation reports.* http://oie.int/en/solidarity/pvs-evaluation-reports/. Accessed 22 July 2019.

PETS ACT. (2006). Pets Evacuation and Transportation Standards; (PETS) Act, S. 2548 and H.R. 3858 2006.

Standring, W. J. F., Dowdall, M., & Strand, P. (2009). Overview of dose assessment developments and the health of riverside residents close to the "Mayak" PA facilities, Russia. *International Journal of Environmental Research and Public Health, 6*(1), 174–199.

UNISDR. (2005). *Hyogo framework for action 2005–2015 building the resilience of nations and communities to disasters.* https://www.unisdr.org/files/1037_hyogoframeworkforactionenglish.pdf

UNISDR. (2015). *Sendai framework for disaster risk reduction 2015–2030.* UNISDR/GE/2015 – ICLUX EN5000 1st edition. https://www.unisdr.org/files/43291_sendaiframeworkfordrren.pdf

USSR Ministry of Agriculture. (1977). *Recommendations on agriculture in the conditions of radioactive contamination of the territory.* "Kolos" 1977 (In Russian).

Vroegindewey, G. (2014). *Animal health in light of natural disasters and bioterrorism.* 2014 – Europe – OIE Regional Commission Proceedings. http://www.oie.int/fileadmin/Home/eng/Publications_%26_Documentation/docs/pdf/TT/2014_EUR1_Vroegindewey_A.pdf

2

Basic Radiobiology

Viktar S. Averyn

2.1 Atoms and Isotopes

The atoms are built up of a nucleus, containing positive (protons) and neutral (neutrons) particles, surrounded by negative particles (electrons), circulating around the "atomic orbit". The number of the protons in the nucleus is giving the atomic number of the element (usually labelled as "Z"), and the sum of the neutrons and protons in the nucleus is giving the atomic or mass number of the element (usually labelled as "A"). The number in the electrons in the atomic orbit is always equal to the number of protons in the nucleus. However, as the mass of the electrons is almost equal to zero, they do not influence the whole atomic mass.

The atomic number and the mass number are defining the properties of the atoms. The oxygen, for example, has eight protons and eight neutrons in the nucleus. If oxygen would have seven protons and seven neutrons, it would be nitrogen. The description of the atomic and mass numbers for atoms or isotopes in the periodic system is expressed by convention as shown in Fig. 2.1.

Some of the atoms have the same number of protons but different number of neutrons. Accordingly, their atomic number will be the same, but the mass number will be greater for the difference in the number of neutrons. These atoms are called **isotopes**. Isotopes, by their nature, can be stable (they do not decay) or, more often, unstable. A schematic example of the hydrogen isotopes deuterium and tritium is given in Fig. 2.2.

An example of the difference between atoms and their respective isotopes is shown in Table 2.1.

V. S. Averyn (✉)
Faculty of Biology, Francisk Skorina Gomel State University, Gomel, Belarus

mass number ⬚	⬚	A ⬚ ⬚
⬚ X	⬚	⬚ X ⬚
atomic number ⬚	neutron number	Z ⬚ N

Fig. 2.1 The mass number (A) is the sum of protons and neutrons in the nucleus of the atom, the atomic number (Z) is the number of protons in the nucleus and the neutron number is labelled as N. From practical reasons, atoms and isotopes are labelled only with A and Z numbers. The N number can be calculated as difference between A and Z (N = A–Z)

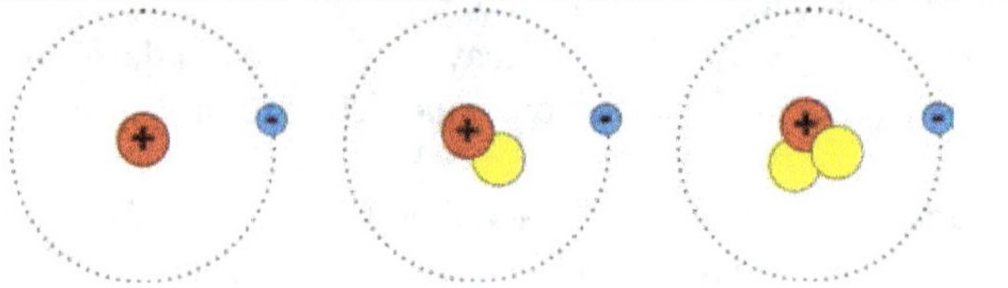

Hydrogen: one proton (red) and one electron (blue)

Deuterium: one proton (red), one neutron (yellow) and one electron (blue)

Tritium: one proton (red), two neutrons (yellow) and one electron (blue)

Fig. 2.2 Schematic example of the hydrogen isotopes deuterium and tritium. (Adapted from IAEA 2004)

Table 2.1 Difference between atoms and isotopes

Number of:	Atoms				Isotopes *			
	$^{1}_{1}H$	$^{12}_{6}C$	$^{14}_{7}N$	$^{16}_{8}O$	$^{2}_{1}H$	$^{13}_{6}C$	$^{15}_{7}N$	$^{18}_{8}O$
Protons (Z)	1	6	7	8	1	6	7	8
Neutrons (N)	**0**	**6**	**7**	**8**	**1**	**7**	**8**	**10**
Mass number (A)	**1**	**12**	**14**	**16**	**2**	**13**	**15**	**18**

*Note the different number of neutrons in the atoms (blue font) and their respective stable isotopes (red font)

2.2 Definition of Radiation

Radiation in its wider definition refers to the energy emitted from various sources of the whole electromagnetic spectrum, such as heat, ultraviolet and visible light, microwaves, radio waves, x-rays, low-frequency radiation (such as used in alternate electric transmission, ultrasound thermal radiation) and ionizing radiation.

The ionizing radiation is the energy emitted from the atomic or subatomic structures in a form of waves (γ rays) or particles (α or ß), as a result of the instability of the isotopes. With the increase of the atomic and mass number, the neutron-to-proton ratio increases, leading to formation of unstable isotopes or so-called "excited" state of the nucleus. Such isotopes tend to reach the "ground" state through the release of α, ß, or γ ionizing radiation (IAEA/WHO 2002).

2.3 Types of Ionizing Radiation

Alpha (α) particles (α decay, α radioactivity) are produced when two neutrons and two protons (i.e. the nucleus of helium) are released from an excited nucleus of the isotopes with higher mass numbers ($Z > 83$, such as uranium, thorium and radium), as shown schematically in Fig. 2.3.

Therefore, the consequence of the α decay is decreased in the atomic number of the resulting decay (daughter) isotope by 2 and decrease in the mass number by 4 (Fig. 2.4).

The alpha particles are positively charged and because of their large mass (4), they cannot penetrate deep in the body. They can reach a distance of few centimetres through open air and cannot penetrate a sheet of paper. However, once entered in the body, usually by inhalation (lungs) or ingestion GI tract, they may cause short range but devastating consequences for the cell's structures (IAEA 2004). An example of alpha decay is shown in Fig. 2.5.

Beta (ß) particles (ß decay, ß radioactivity) are generated when the nucleus of an isotope has too many protons or neutrons (neutron or proton deficiency, respectively) and are the result of the tendency of the nucleus to rearrange itself to a more stable configuration. Consequently, there are two types of ß decay, the β^- and β^+ decay.

2.3.1 *β^- Decay*

In case when the nucleus has too many neutrons (it is proton deficient), the neutrons (n) are converted to protons (p) by releasing an electron (β^- particle), under high speed (approximately the speed of light) and a particle without mass and charge, called anti-neutrino ($\tilde{\nu}$). The changes during β^- decay may be described as follows:

$n \rightarrow p + \beta^- + \tilde{\nu}$ (Fig. 2.6)

Thus, during β^- decay, the atomic number of the resulting decay (daughter) isotope increases for 1, while the mass number remains the same (Fig. 2.7).

An example of β^- decay is shown in Fig. 2.8.

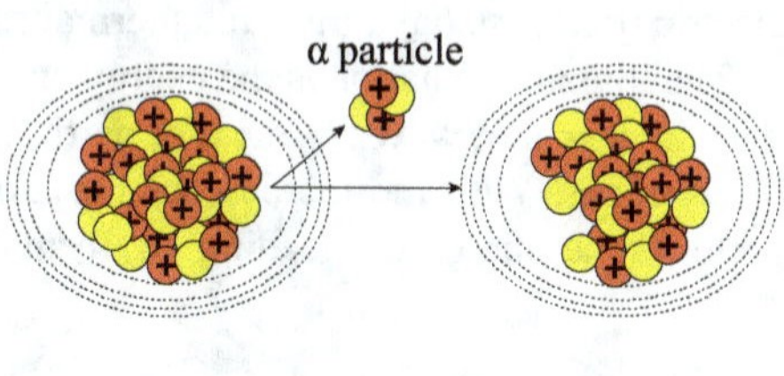

Fig. 2.3 Schematic example of α decay. (Adapted from IAEA/WHO 2002)

$$^{A}_{Z}X \xrightarrow[\text{decay}]{\alpha} {}^{A-4}_{Z-2}Y$$

Fig. 2.4 General pattern of the changes in the atomic and the mass number of the resulting decay product (Y) from the source isotope (X) during α decay

$$^{241}_{95}Am \xrightarrow[\text{decay}]{\alpha} {}^{237}_{93}Np$$

Americium 241 → Neptunium 237

Fig. 2.5 Examples of an α decay are shown in following examples. *Note: the decrease in the atomic and the mass number of the resulting daughter isotopes (blue font) compared to the respective numbers of the decaying parent isotope (red fonts)

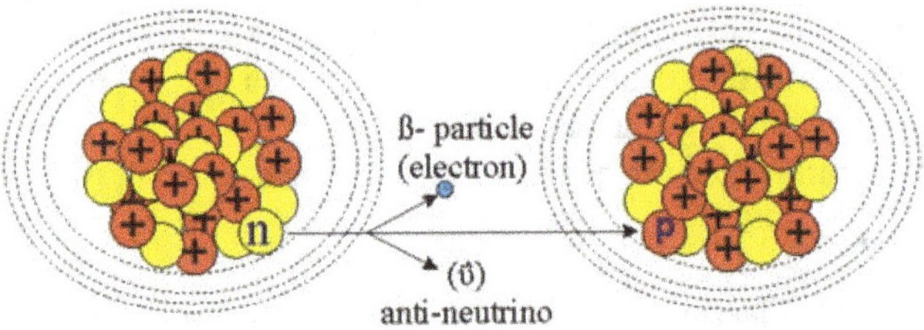

Fig. 2.6 Schematic example of ß⁻decay. Note the change of the yellow-filled neutron (n) to a red-filled proton (p), following the long arrow. (Adapted from IAEA/WHO 2002)

$$^{A}_{Z}X \xrightarrow{\beta^{-}\text{ decay}} {}^{A}_{Z+1}Y$$

Fig. 2.7 General pattern of the changes in the atomic number of the resulting daughter product (Y) from the source parent isotope (X) during ß⁻ decay

$$^{131}_{53}I \xrightarrow{\beta^{-}\text{ decay}} {}^{131}_{54}Xe$$

Iodine 131 → Xenon 131

Fig. 2.8 Example of a ß⁻ decay of ^{131}I to ^{131}Xe. *Note the increase of the atomic number by maintaining the same mass number of the resulting daughter isotope (blue font) compared to the respective numbers of the decaying parent isotope (red fonts)

2.3.2 *β^+ Decay*

In case when the nucleus has too many protons (it is neutron deficient), the protons (p) are converted to neutrons (n) by releasing a positron (positively charged electron, β^+ particle), under high speed (approximately the speed of light) and a particle without mass and charge, called neutrino (υ). The changes during β^+ decay may be described as follows:

$p \rightarrow n + \beta^+ + \upsilon$ (Fig. 2.9)

Thus, during β^+ decay, the atomic number of the resulting decay (daughter) isotope decreases for 1, while the mass number remains the same (Fig. 2.10).

An example of β^+ decay is shown in Fig. 2.11.

2.3.3 *Electron Capture*

In case when the nucleus has protons in excess (situation similar to the β^+ decay), the protons (p) may be converted to neutrons (n) by the phenomenon called electron capture. In such cases, the orbital electrons are captured by the protons which convert to neutrons by emitting a neutrino (υ).

The changes during electron capture may be described as follows:

$p + e \rightarrow n + \upsilon$ (Fig. 2.12)

Thus, during the electron capture (similar as during the β^+ decay), the atomic number of the resulting decay (daughter) isotope decreases for 1, while the mass number remains the same (Fig. 2.13). An example of electron capture is shown in Fig. 2.14.

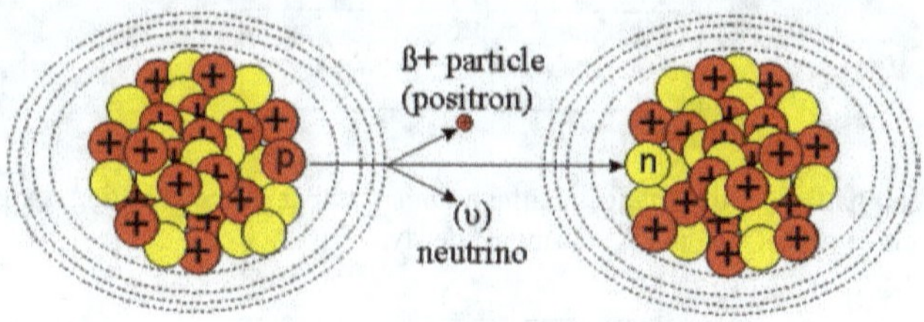

Fig. 2.9 Schematic example of β^+ decay. Note the change of the red-filled proton (p) to a yellow-filled neutron (n), following the long arrow. (Adapted from IAEA/WHO 2002)

$${}^{A}_{Z}X \xrightarrow{\beta^+ \text{ decay}} {}^{\;\;\;\;A}_{Z-1}Y$$

Fig. 2.10 General pattern of the changes in the atomic number of the resulting decay product (Y) from the source isotope (X) during β^+ decay

$$^{18}_{9}\mathrm{F} \xrightarrow{\beta^+ \text{ decay}} {}^{18}_{8}\mathrm{O}$$

Fluorine 18 → *Oxygen 18*

Fig. 2.11 Example of a ß⁺ decay of ^{18}F to ^{18}O. *Note the decrease of the atomic number by maintaining the same mass number of the resulting daughter isotope (blue font) compared to the respective numbers of the decaying parent isotope (red fonts)

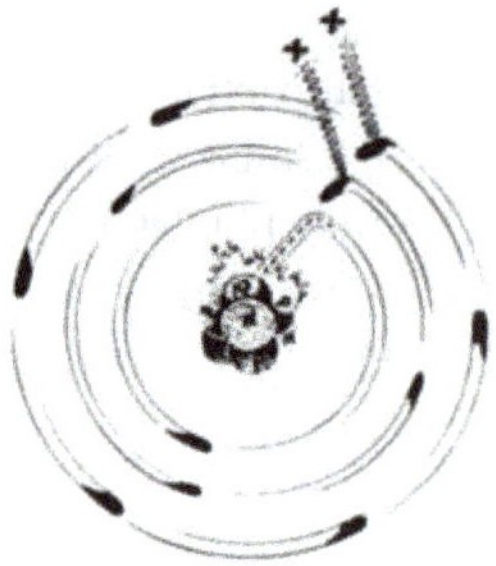

Fig. 2.12 Schematic example of the electron capture. Note the orbital electron is captured by the proton from the nucleus. (From IAEA/WHO 2002)

$$^{A}_{Z}\mathrm{X} \xrightarrow{\text{Electron Capture}} {}^{A}_{Z-1}\mathrm{Y}$$

Fig. 2.13 General pattern of the changes in the atomic number of the resulting decay product (Y) from the source isotope (X) during electron capture

$$^{125}_{53}\mathrm{I} \xrightarrow{\text{electron capture}} {}^{125}_{52}\mathrm{Te}$$

Iodine 125 → *Tellurium 125*

Fig. 2.14 Example of an electron capture of the ^{125}I to ^{125}Te. *Note: the decrease of the atomic number by maintaining the same mass number of the resulting daughter isotope (blue font) compared to the respective numbers of the decaying parent isotope (red fonts). (From IAEA/WHO 2002)

During the electron capture, specific x-rays are emitted, and, in some cases, where an excess of energy remains, γ rays are also emitted (IAEA/WHO 2002).

Gamma (γ) rays (γ radioactivity) are high-energy electromagnetic rays (similar to x-rays) which are produced in the atomic nucleus. They have no electrical charge and an extremely high frequency (over 10^{19} Hz) and energy (over 100 keV). For this reason, they have highly penetrating potential. Their release may be induced through excitation of the atomic nucleus by other decay processes, such as α or ß decay (Fig. 2.15).

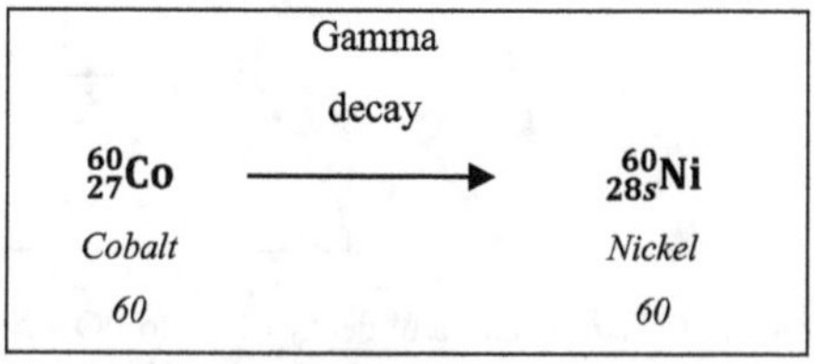

Fig. 2.15 Example of gamma decay of the ^{60}Co to ^{60}Ni

2.4 Physical Half-Life of Radioactive Isotopes

Each radioactive isotope, by emission of certain particles and/or rays, expends the energy (radioactivity) and tends towards stabilization. The time required to expend half of the radioactivity is called physical half-life of the radioactive isotope and is most commonly labelled as $T_{1/2}$. Each isotope has specific physical half-life; thus the calculation of $T_{1/2}$ is based on the isotope constant, as follows:

$$T_{1/2} = \text{Ln}\,2 / \lambda$$

where λ is a radioactive constant specific for the isotope.

Very often, it is necessary to predict the activity of certain isotope, after a certain time (A). This can be also calculated, based on the initial radioactivity (A_0), the isotope constant (λ) and the elapsed period (t), as follows:

$$A = A_0 + e^{(-\lambda t)},$$

where the "e" is the natural logarithm and has the value of 271,828.

A list of the most important isotopes, the ionizing particles/rays are emitting, and the physical half-lives are shown in Table 2.2. The schematic overview of the radioactive decay of isotopes with short (^{131}I, 8 days), long (^{137}Cs, 30 years) and very long (^{239}Pu, 24,390 years) half-life is shown in Fig. 2.16.

2.5 Biological Half-Life of the Radioactive Isotopes

Once entered into the body of animals, via the intestines or inhalation, a part of the ingested radionuclides is absorbed into the blood stream, and the rest is excreted via the faeces or exhaled. The amount entered into the blood stream is distributed among the different tissues. The distribution pathways vary for different isotopes. Some isotopes are distributed throughout the body, and some are incorporated into certain organs. Absorbed radionuclides can be excreted in urine or endogenously excreted in the faeces. The time required for a radioactive isotope to lose half of its activity in the body is called the biological half-life ($T^{b}_{1/2}$) which depends on the metabolic characteristics of each isotope and is not related to the physical half-life of the isotope ($T^{p}_{1/2}$). Some of the isotopes may have short $T_{1/2}$ and long $T^{b}_{1/2}$, and the opposite also occurs.

Table 2.2 List of most important radioisotopes, occurring after a NRE, their mass number, type of decay and the physical half-life

Radioactive element	Atomic number	Atomic mass number	Decay type	Half-life
Cesium (Cs)	**55**	**134**	**(β-), γ**	**2 years**
Cesium (Cs)	55	135	(β-), γ	2 million years
Cesium (Cs)	**55**	**137**	**(β-), γ**	**30 years**
Iodine (I)	53	129	(β-), γ	17.2×10^6 years
Iodine (I)	**53**	**131**	**(β-), γ**	**8 days**
Iodine (I)	53	134	(β-), γ	52 min
Plutonium (Pu)	94	236	α	285 years
Plutonium (Pu)	94	238	α	86 years
Plutonium (Pu)	**94**	**239**	**α**	**24,390 years**
Plutonium (Pu)	94	240	α	6580 years
Plutonium (Pu)	94	241	(β-), α	13 years
Plutonium (Pu)	94	242	α	379,000 years
Plutonium (Pu)	94	243	α	5 years
Plutonium (Pu)	94	244	α	76×10^6 years
Strontium (Sr)	**38**	**89**	**(β-)**	**53 days**
Strontium (Sr)	**38**	**90**	**(β-)**	**28 years**

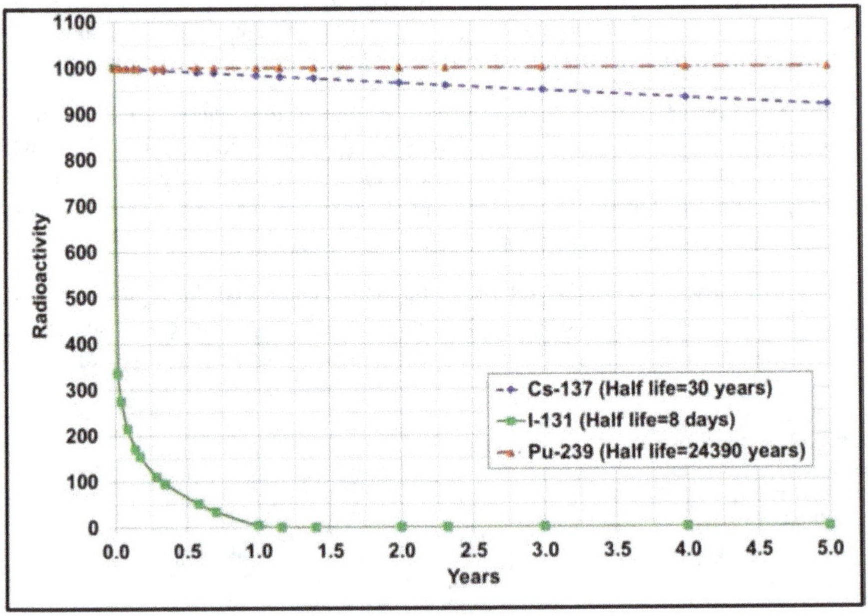

Fig. 2.16 Schematic overview of the radioactive decay of three isotopes with different half-life (simulation of a 5-year period)

2.6 Effective Half-Life of the Radioactive Isotopes in the Body of Animals

The effective half-life ($T_{1/2}^{\text{eff}}$) is the time required to lose half of the overall activity in the body and is a result of the interrelation between the $T_{1/2}^{p}$ and $T_{1/2}^{b}$. The $T_{1/2}^{\text{eff}}$ can be calculated according to the following equation:

$$T_{1/2}^{\text{eff}} = \left(T_{1/2}^{p} \times T_{1/2}^{b}\right) / \left(T_{1/2}^{p} + T_{1/2}^{b}\right)$$

Example: Iodine-131 has a $T_{1/2}^{p}$ of 8 days and a $T_{1/2}^{b}$ of 138 days. The $T_{1/2}^{\text{eff}}$ can be calculated as:

$$T_{1/2}^{\text{eff}} = (8 \times 138) / (8 + 138) = 1104 / 146 = 7.6\,\text{days}.$$

2.7 Decay Chains and Ingrowth

The radioactive isotopes undergo radioactive decay through numerous transformations. Until the last decay, with each transformation, these radionuclides emit particles (energy) and become another isotope (Fig. 2.17). This stepwise decay ends with formation of a stable atom or isotope and is called decay chain of the specific isotope.

The result of the decay chain is a dynamic change of the concentration of different between-products (isotopes); unit of the final stable product is formed. Through this process, the concentration of the source nucleotide continuously decreases, and the concentration of between products increases, until the final, stable element achieves the maximal concentration. This process is called ingrowth (Fig. 2.18).

Information and knowledge related to the decay chain and the ingrowth are of utmost importance for the waste management or post-accident mitigation strategies, even though some of these processes may continue over thousands of years!

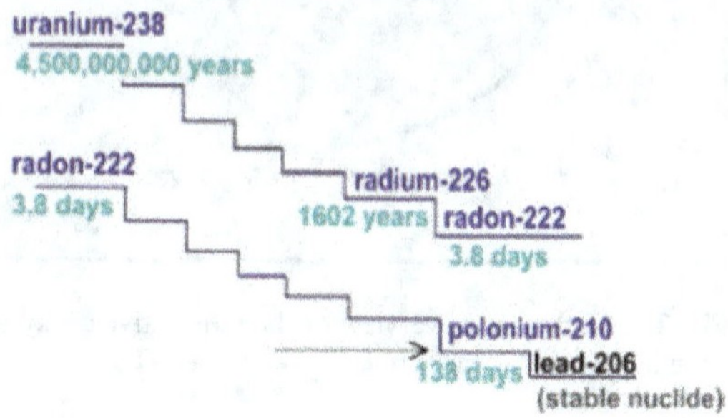

Fig. 2.17 Example of a decay chain for unstable (radioactive) ^{238}U to stable lead (EPA 2015a)

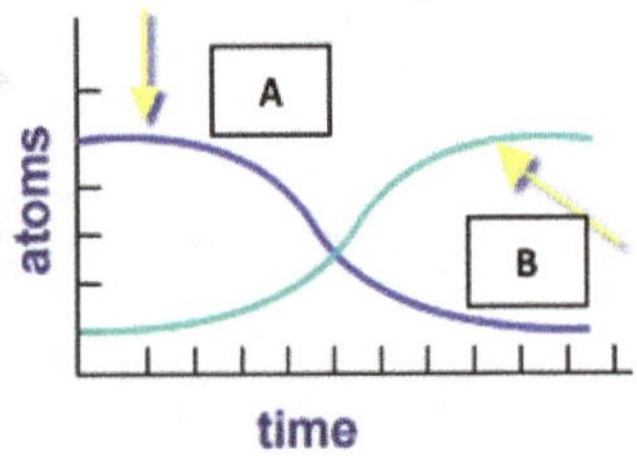

Fig. 2.18 As decay progresses, the concentration of original radionuclide is decreasing (A), while the concentration of the stable decay product is increasing! (EPA 2015b)

There are three natural (uranium, thorium and actinium) and one artificial (americium) decay series, for which detailed information on the type of radiation, energy and half-lives of parent and daughter isotopes are calculated (US Department of Energy 1997). Detailed calculation of the decay and growth of individual parent and daughter isotopes, respectively, is given in IAEA/UNESCO (2000).

2.8 Units of Radioactivity

The radioactivity of the isotopes represents decays per time unit. According to the SI system, the measure for radioactivity is Becquerel (Bq) and represents one disintegration per second. The conventional unit, Curie (Ci), has been defined as activity of 1 g of ^{226}Ra (IAEA 2004) and equals 37×10^9 disintegrations per second. Accordingly, 1 Ci = 3.7×10^{10} Bq or 1 Ci = 3.7 GBq and 1 Bq = 2.703×10^{-11} Ci.

2.9 Specific Radioactivity

Specific radioactivity is the radioactivity per mass or volume of certain material. It is expressed as Bq/kg (mass) or Bq/m^3 (volume). The legislation limits for animal products are based on the specific radioactivity.

2.10 Radiation Dose

The radiation dose is the amount of radiation energy (amount of radiation exposures) absorbed by the body and is defined by two variables:

The absorbed dose (physical dose) is the amount of energy deposited in a unit of mass in the tissue or other media. The SI unit for absorbed dose is Gray (Gy) and represents an energy of 1 Joule/kg mass. In older literature, Rad is used, which is 100 times smaller dose than Gray (1 Gray = 100 Rad).

The dose equivalent (biological dose) takes into consideration the total energy deposited and the amount of energy lost from the particles (rays) per unit dis-

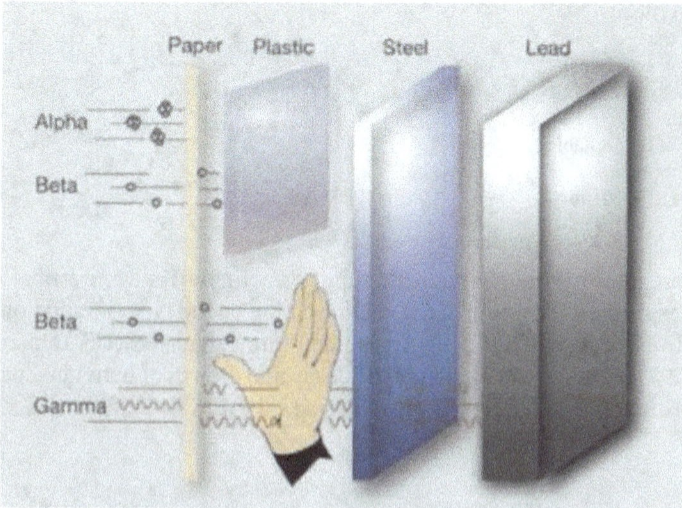

Fig. 2.19 A schematic example of the capacity for penetration of α and β particles and γ rays through different materials (IAEA 2004)

tance (linear energy transfer or LET). The LET depends on the size of the particles, their charge and their energy. Larger and charged particles (α and β) have higher LET compared to γ rays. Schematic example of the capacity for penetration of the ionizing radiation through different substances is shown in Fig. 2.19.

The biological effect of different radiation particles/rays is measured by the quality factor (Q). The Q factor is a correction for different types of radiation particles/rays, used to correct for the biological effect caused by these particles. For electrons, x-rays and gamma rays, the Q is taken to be 1; for alpha particles it is 20 and for neutrons varies from 5 to 20, depending on neutron energy (Table 2.3). The biological impact is specified by the dose equivalent (H), which is the product of the absorbed dose D and the quality factor (Radiation weighting factors) Q (H = QxD). Consequently, if an organism has absorbed a dose of 1 Gy of gamma rays, the dose equivalent would be 1 Sv, whereas for the same absorbed dose of alpha particles, the dose equivalent would be 20 Sv. In older literature, instead of Sievert, the Rem unit is used, which is a product of Rads × Q. The Sievert is 100 times higher than the Rem (1 Sv = 100 Rem).

2.11 Effective Dose Equivalent

Even if same biological dose is absorbed by different organs or biological systems, the overall risk may vary depending on the organ/biological system affected. The effective dose equivalent is therefore discounted for the appropriate weighting factor, in order to reflect the overall risk. Estimated weighting factors for some parts of the body are shown in Table 2.4.

Table 2.3 The quality factors (Q) of different types of ionizing (Gusev et al. 2001)

Body part	Quality factors
Protons (all energies)	1
Electrons (all energies)	1
Neutrons (<10 keV)	5
(<10–100 keV)	10
(100 keV–2 MeV)	20
(2–20 MeV)	10
(>20 MeV)	5
Protons (>2 MeV)	5
Alpha particles, fission fragments, heavy nuclei	20

Table 2.4 The estimated weighting factors for selected organs of the human body (ICRP 2012)

Body part	Weighting factor
Whole body	1 (100%)
Ovaria, testis	0.25 (25%)
Bone marrow	0.12 (12%)
Bone surface	0.03 (3%)
Thyroid gland	0.03 (3%)
Chest	0.15 (15%)
Lungs	0.12 (12%)
Other tissues	0.3 (30%)

2.12 Lethal Dose

The effective dose equivalent that will cause death in 50% of the exposed individuals is called 50% lethal dose (LD_{50}), and it is different for different species.

LD50 in different animal species is shown in Table 2.5.

A simplified way for interpretation of the units of radiation mentioned above is shown in Table 2.6.

2.13 Interaction of the Ionizing Radiation with the Matter

Based on their mass and the energy of the ionizing radiation, different sources have different capacities of penetration through the matter. They have also different biological action when entered into the body of humans and animals.

During penetration, the ionizing particles are causing electrical interactions with the matter, either by interactions with the electrons (α, β and γ) or interactions with the atomic nuclei (neutrons). The energy that is lost during the penetration of the ionizing radiation causes vibrations of the atomic and molecular structures, which results in short heat production in biological tissues. Ionization and the consequent

Table 2.5 LD 50% for different animal species (Gy) (Yarmonenko 1988)

Species	Dose (Gy)	Species	Dose (Gy)
Sheep	1.5–2.5	Birds	8.0–20.0
Donkey	2.0–3.8	Fishes	8.0–20.0
Dog	2.5–3.0	Rabbit	9.0–10.0
Monkeys (different species)	2.5–6.0	Hamster	9.0–10.0
Mice (different lines)	6.0–15.0	Snake	80.0–200.0
		Plants	10.0–1500.0

Table 2.6 Illustration of simplified ways of interpretation of different units for measuring radiation exposure (Gusev et al. 2001)

Amount of radioactivity	Quantity	Unit
How much radioactivity is in the observed matrix (sample)	Specific radioactivity	Bq/kg
How much radioactivity (energy) has been deposited (for human population only)	Absorbed dose	Gy
Deposited energy (absorbed dose) corrected for the quality factor of the radiation type (alpha, beta, gamma)	Equivalent (biological) dose	Sv
Effective dose, corrected for the weighting factor of the organ (tissue) affected	Effective dose equivalent	Sv

chemical changes are actually the reason for the harmful biological effects of the ionizing radiation (IAEA 2004).

2.14 The Sources of Man-Made Environmental Contamination

Continuous nuclear tests (UNSCEAR 1977), radiation accidents and large-scale nuclear disasters (Dyachenko 2008) have led to the omnipresent pollution of the biosphere by radioactive hazardous substances such as ^{137}Cs and ^{90}Sr. Nowadays, the typical density of land contamination caused by these radionuclides makes up a few tens of kBq/m^2.

Four hundred twenty-three nuclear explosions were conducted in the atmosphere during the period of nuclear testing in 1945–1980. Altogether, they discharged around 5.9×19^{17} Bq of ^{90}Sr and approximately 9.5×10^{17} Bq of ^{137}Cs. The present-time deposition density of these radionuclides in the mid-latitudes of the Northern Hemisphere, from both nuclear testing and global fallouts, makes up 1.1 and 1.8 kBq/m^2, respectively.

The radiation accident of 27 September 1957 that had occurred at "Mayak" reprocessing nuclear facility in Chelyabinsk region, USSR, involved the explosion of 70–80 tons of high-activity nuclear wastes with a total activity of around 7.4×10^{17} Bq, of which approximately 7.4×10^{16} Bq was released into the environment. The contribution of ^{90}Sr and ^{137}Cs in the total discharged activity was 2×10^{15} and 3×10^{13} Bq, respectively. The extensive radioactive trace with a total area over 1000 km^2 and ^{90}Sr contamination level of 74 kBq/m^2 had spread over USSR's Chelyabinsk, Sverdlovsk and Tyumen regions (Aleksakhin 2006; Avramenko et al. 1997).

On 26 April 1986, the radiation disaster at the Chernobyl NPP was accompanied by powerful releases of radioactive materials into the atmosphere. The total activity of radioactive materials released from the nuclear core in the accident was $(1–2) \times 10^{18}$ Bq, with a share of ^{137}Cs equalling to 3.6×10^{16} Bq and that of ^{90}Sr equalling to 8.0×10^{15} Bq (IAEA 2008).

Two hundred sixty-five thousand hectares of the agricultural lands in Belarus are contaminated by either ^{137}Cs or and ^{90}Sr with the deposition densities of above 1480 kBq/m^2 and 111 kBq/m^2, respectively (CMRB 1997). A particular challenge for the country has been the production of foods in compliance with the regulation values in the areas where land contamination by cesium-137 is 5–40 Ci/km^2. The total area of such lands in the republic is 415.6 thousand hectares, of which 35.7 thousand hectares is simultaneously contaminated by ^{90}Sr with a density of 1–3 Ci/km^2 (Annenkov and Averin 2003).

The most important and equally complicated task of the regional development strategy is about overcoming the consequences of the Chernobyl disaster. The strategy of sustainable development of the areas affected by radioactive contamination should be built with taking into account the need to improve the living standards and the overall wellbeing of the residents on the basis of environmentally radiological and socio-economic recovery of such areas. The following efforts are planned to help to reach this objective:

- Reduction of poverty and unemployment, increased profits, enhancement of social protection of affected populations based on revival of economic activities in affected areas, intensification of investment projects, creation of favourable conditions for the development of farming, small and medium businesses
- Improvement of living conditions, social and cultural environments of the residents of affected areas, particularly in the countryside

References

Aleksakhin, R. M. (2006). *Problems of radioecology: Evolution of ideas. The results*. M. Russian Agricultural Academy. GNU VNIISKHRAE, 880 p.

Annenkov, B. N., & Averin V. S. (2003). *Agriculture in areas of radioactive contamination (radionuclides in foodstuffs)*. Mn: Propylene, pp. 111c.

Avramenko, M. I., et. al. (1997). *The 1957 accident. Evolution of explosion parameters and analysis of the terrestrial radioactive contamination characteristics issues*. Radiat. Saf. N3, pp. 18–29 (In Russian).

CMRB. (1997). Resolution of the Council of Ministers of the Republic of Belarus (CMRB) of 27.03.1997 N 255 “On the National Strategy for the Sustainable Development of the Republic of Belarus”.

Dyachenko, A. A. (2008). *Scorched in the struggle during the creation of the nuclear shield of the Motherland* (V. N. Mikhailov, Ed.). M. Polygraph-Service, 596 p.

EPA. (2015a). *Environmental Protection Agency – Radioactive decay*. https://www.epa.gov/radiation/radioactive-decay

EPA. (2015b). *Environmental Protection Agency – Ingrowth*. http://www.epa.gov/radiation/understand/chain.html

Gusev, I., Guskova, A., & Mettler, F. (Eds.). (2001). *Medical management of radiological accidents*. CRC Press LLC. ISBN: 0-8493-7004-3.

IAEA. (2004). *Radiation, people and the environment*. https://www.iaea.org/sites/default/files/radiation0204.pdf

IAEA. (2008). *Ecological consequences of the chernobyl accident and their overcoming: Twenty years of experience*. Report of the Ecology expert group of the IAEA Chernobyl Forum, p. 94.

IAEA/UNESCO. (2000). *Environmental isotopes in hydrological cycle*. http://www-naweb.iaea.org/napc/ih/documents/global_cycle/Environmental%20Isotopes%20in%20the%20Hydrological%20Cycle%20Vol%201.pdf

IAEA/WHO. (2002). *Medical preparedness and response*. EPRMEDICAL/T 2002. Available at: http://www-pub.iaea.org/MTCD/publications/PDF/eprmedt/Start.pdf

ICRP. (2012). *Compendium of dose coefficients based on ICRP Publication 60*. http://www.icrp.org/docs/P%20119%20JAICRP%2041(s)%20Compendium%20of%20Dose%20Coefficients%20based%20on%20ICRP%20Publication%2060.pdf

UNSCEAR. (1977). *Sources and effects of ionizing radiation*. UN Scientific Committee on the Effects of Atomic Radiation 1977 Report to the General Assembly with Attachments, Vol. 1, United Nations, New York, 1978, 381 p.

US Department of Energy. (1997). HASL-300, 28th Edition, Section 5, Vol. 1: Radionuclide data. https://www.wipp.energy.gov/namp/emllegacy/ProcMan/sections/SECT5.PDF

Yarmonenko, S. P. (1988). *Radiobiology of humans and animals*. Moscow: Mir Publishers. ISBN: 5030000623, 9785030000626.

3

Radiation Measuring Instruments

Viktar S. Averyn

3.1 Measuring Instruments

Three basic types of measuring instruments used for the purposes of radiation control and monitoring are spectrometers, radiometers and dosimeters (Gurachevsky 2010).

Spectrometers (Fig. 3.1) provide the most complete information about radiation. The most frequently used ones are spectrometers for measuring gamma-ray spectra. They are equipped with semiconductor or scintillation detectors that have high-energy resolution. The most informative part of the gamma-spectrum from the particular radionuclide is the total absorption peak. Its position is determined by the energy of gamma-radiation, and its height – by the intensity. In this manner, spectrometers are used for both qualitative and quantitative analyses of the content of the sample as they can determine not only the composition of radionuclides in the sample but also their activities. The role of processing the spectra is usually played by personal computers.

In measuring radiation from beta- and alpha-particles, because of their low penetrating power, the layer of the sample closest to the detector contributes to the detected radiation. Penetration of radiation should not be obstructed by the walls of a sample vessel placed inside the detector or because of the walls of its entrance window. This interference can be totally avoided by dissolving a sample in the liquid scintillator.

To enhance sensitivity of the measuring device, the samples are preprocessed using a thermal scavenging technique to the point of being partially ashed. Liquid samples, e.g. water or milk, are first filtered through fibrous cationites, then dried and used as samples.

V. S. Averyn (✉)
Faculty of Biology, Francisk Skorina Gomel State University , Gomel, Belarus

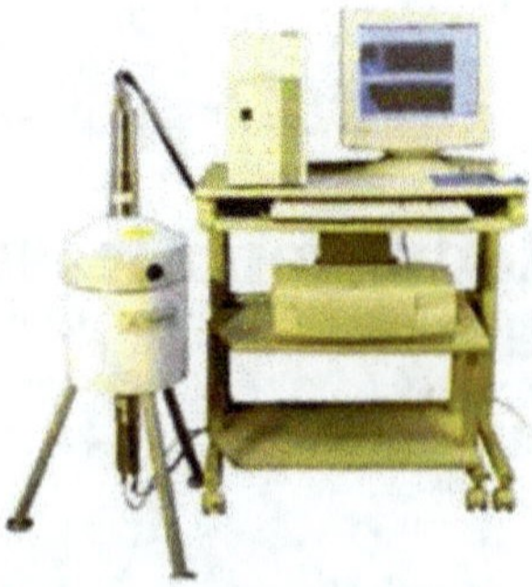

Fig. 3.1 Gamma-beta spectrometer. (From: Gurachevsky 2010)

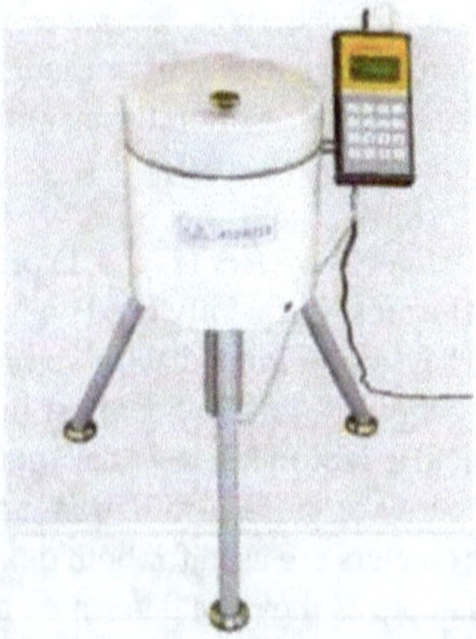

Fig. 3.2 Gamma-radiometer. (From: Gurachevsky 2010)

The most complicated spectrometers are alpha-spectrometers. Since alpha-radiation has a very low penetrating ability, the measurements are typically carried out in a vacuum chamber using a semiconductor detector. Importantly, the composition of radionuclides is determined by measuring "thin" samples placed on special plates using a technique called electrode position. The total activity, on the other hand, is a much easier task, since it can be determined by measuring "thick" samples obtained through attrition and chemical or thermal concentration methods.

The main purpose of radiometers is measuring the specific activity and activity concentration (volumetric activity) of the sources of ionizing radiation. The most commonly used are radiometers for measuring gamma-emitting radionuclides.

The simplest radiometers are able to determine activity by counting all detector pulses with the deduction of the background with account for the geometry. However, the most efficient radiometers are those with discriminative characteristics which can offer selective properties to react only to radiations emitted from a particular radionuclide. Such partition becomes possible due to the built-in electronic circuits able of selecting detector signals of certain amplitudes and a microprocessor for data processing. Modern-day radiometers, such as RKG-AT1320 (Fig. 3.2), are just like a downsized version of spectrometers.

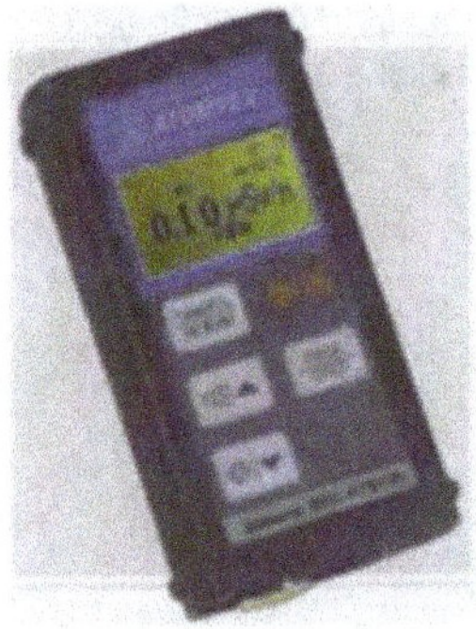

Fig. 3.3 X-ray and gamma-radiation dosimeter. (From: Gurachevsky 2010)

Whole-body counters (WBC), used for measuring the activity of ^{137}Cs in a human body, can also be classified as radiometers. A typical WBC has a chair equipped with several scintillation detectors intended for different parts of the body. Using the resulting readings, one can assess the internal radiation dose of a person. The WBC for measuring the content of strontium-90 is a considerably more complex device. There are only a few whole-body counters of that kind in the world.

Dosimeters (Fig. 3.3) are aimed at assessing the equivalent or effective radiation doses. The simplest devices are suited only to be able to detect photon radiations, i.e. gamma- and X-rays. A typical dosimeter is built using inexpensive Geiger-Mueller counters, the signals of which do not yield information about the photon energy. Diverse contribution into the absorbed dose made by the photons of different energy levels is taken into account by adjusting the energy response through filter compensation.

3.1.1 Personnel Dosimeters

Personnel exposed to ionizing radiation are monitored to determine their occupational exposure. Although this consists primarily of monitoring external exposure, it is also necessary to assess the need to monitor internal exposure and, if necessary, incorporate it into a worker's total monitoring system. External monitoring can be accomplished by using photographic film or thermoluminescent or pocket dosimeters (Fig. 3.4).

3.2 Measuring Contamination Levels in Live Farm Animals

Animal products represent as a major contributor to the internal dose, and live monitoring of animals is an integral part of many remedial actions. Radiocaesium can be measured in live animals using a robust gamma-monitor applied to the muscle mass of a restrained animal. Live monitoring is a rapid, simple, inexpensive and effective

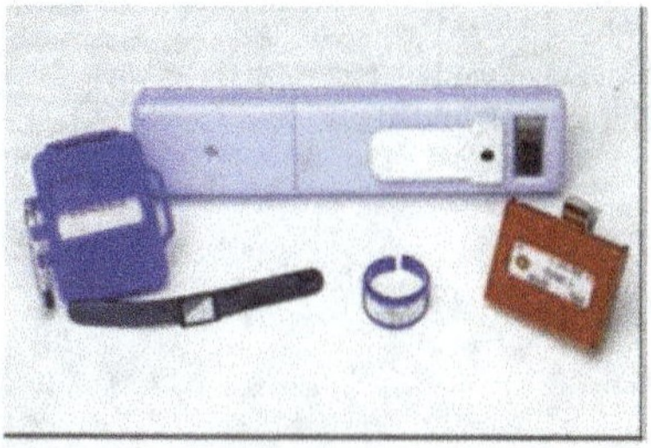

Fig. 3.4 Different types of pocket dosimeters. (From: Gurachevsky 2010)

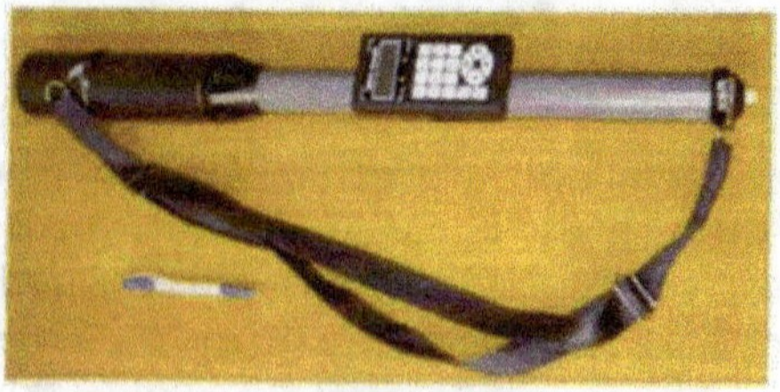

Fig. 3.5 MKS-01 Sovetnik. (From: Gurachevsky 2010)

method of monitoring contamination for gamma-emitting radionuclides. The monitoring needs to be conducted using a robust and portable, preferably lead-shielded, NaI detector, linked to (or with integral) single or multichannel analysers (RIARAE 1993; Brynilsen and Strand 1994). In areas of elevated external dose, it may be necessary to ensure adequate shielding to attain sufficiently low minimum detachable levels in the detector. Live monitoring of livestock is largely relevant for gamma-emitters, notably radiocaesium. It can be carried out on the farm and also at slaughterhouses. These measurements are performed largely before slaughtering to confirm that intervention levels are not exceeded.

Some dosimeters, e.g. a modern device MKS-AT6130 (Fig. 3.3), can detect the flux density of beta-rays from the contaminated surface. In this mode, the filter-equipped lid, hinged on special joints, is flicked open. Since the flux density measurement is typically related to radiometry objectives, such devices are called dosimeters-radiometers.

Another multipurpose instrument worth mentioning is the MKS-01 Sovetnik dosimeter-radiometer (Fig. 3.5). It uses a large-volume scintillation detector (196 cm^3) and original algorithms of functioning and information processing.

In its dose measuring mode, Sovetnik has a significantly higher sensitivity as compared to more simplified instruments, with only 2–3 s needed to reach 10% statistical error of the measurement. For this reason, the use of Sovetnik in its "dosimeter" function is very efficient in controlling the homogeneity of the produce batches. As a radiometer, Sovetnik is exceptionally convenient for measuring contamination levels in live farm animals, notably the cattle.

Photographic film dosimeter is sensitive to ionizing radiation, and when it is used as a monitor, the amount of film darkening is a measurement of radiation exposure. The filmstrip and holder constitute the film monitor, called a ***film badge***. This film badge has a small, open window that allows the film to be exposed with most X-ray and gamma-radiation and high-energy beta-radiation. The film badge also contains a set of plastic and metal filters. Since different types and energies of radiation will be attenuated differently by these filters, the pattern on the processed film may be used to determine the type, approximate energy, and intensity of exposure. Since film response is energy dependent, this approximate energy determination allows the use of a film energy response calibration curve. Such monitors can be used for exposures as low as 0.01 mSv and as high as several Sv.

Target of the measurement	Tissue
Level of radioactive contamination – radiation dose rate in area	Portable instruments (survey meters)
Identity and quantity of radioactive material	Laboratory counters
Accumulated dose to individuals in area	Personnel dosimeters

References

Brynilsen, L., & Strand, P. (1994). A rapid method for the determination of radioactive caesium in live animals and carcasses and its practical application in Norway after the chernobyl accident. *Acta Veterinaria Scandinavica, 35*, 401–408.

Gurachevsky, V. L. (2010). *Radiation control: Physical fundamentals and instrumental base: A manual* (166 p). Minsk: Institute of Radiology.

RIARAE. (1993). *Intravital determination of the concentration of cesium-137 in the muscle tissue of farm animals*. All-Union Scientific Research Institute of Agricultural Radiology (RIARAE), Belarusian and Ukrainian Branches, Obninsk 1993. (In Russian).

4

Animal Production Systems: Requirements and Guidelines

Kevin Kelleher

4.1 Relevant IAEA Publications on Emergency Preparedness and Response for Animal Production Systems

The IAEA has published Safety Standards and Scientific and Technical Publications to assist in developing an adequate level of preparedness and response for a NRE and includes:

- General Safety Requirements No. GSR Part 7 – Preparedness and Response for a Nuclear or Radiological Emergency (IAEA 2015)
- General Safety Guide No. GSG-2 – Criteria for Use in Preparedness and Response for a Nuclear or Radiological Emergency (IAEA 2011)
- Safety Guide No. GSG-2.1 – Arrangements for Preparedness for a Nuclear or Radiological Emergency (IAEA 2007a)
- General Safety Guide No. GSG-11 – Arrangements for the Termination of a Nuclear or Radiological Emergency (IAEA 2018a)

This chapter outlines how these requirements and guidelines apply to animal production systems to protect the food chain and water supply, prevent the ingestion of contaminated or potentially contaminated food and protect international trade. The generic criteria at which protective actions and other response actions to be taken in response to a NRE are described and the actions that can be implemented during each phase of any NRE for animal production systems are summarised.

The goals of emergency preparedness and response to a NRE are outlined in the IAEA's General Safety Requirements Part 7 (IAEA 2015). These goals include avoiding or minimising the occurrence of severe health effects due to chronic

K. Kelleher (✉)
Environmental Protection Agency, Dublin, Ireland
e-mail: K.Kelleher@epa.ie

radiation exposure, reducing the risk of stochastic effects (e.g. increased cancer) and mitigation of the consequences of an emergency.

4.2 Phases of a Nuclear or Radiological Emergency

The arrangements, protective actions and other response actions outlined in this publication are implemented at various phases of a nuclear or radiological emergency to ensure there is adequate preparedness and response to a NRE. The stage at which the protective actions and other response actions are implemented is important to ensure their maximum effectiveness in emergency preparedness and response. Figure 4.1 outlines the various phases and exposure situations for a nuclear or radiological emergency. The phases of the emergency exposure situation are defined only for planning purposes to ensure adequate provisions are in place for an effective response in an emergency. However, during the response to a NRE, it is difficult to clearly distinguish between these various phases, especially between the early response phase and transition phase (IAEA 2015).

4.2.1 The Preparedness Stage

The preparedness stage is the stage at which adequate capabilities are in place for an effective emergency response in a nuclear or radiological emergency. This capability consists of a set of elements that include but are not limited to:

- Authority and responsibilities
- Organisation and staffing
- Coordination
- Plans and procedures
- Tools, equipment and facilities
- Training drills and exercises and
- A management system

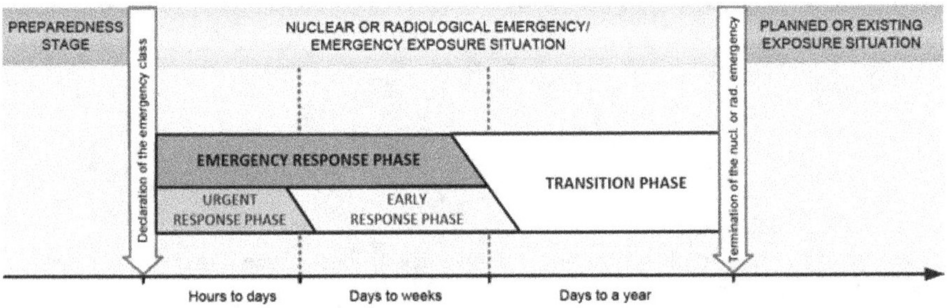

Fig. 4.1 Temporal sequence of the various phases and exposure situations for a nuclear or radiological emergency (IAEA 2018a)

This is the time to ensure an emergency management system is established and maintained and that roles and responsibilities for preparedness and response for a nuclear or radiological emergency are clearly specified and clearly assigned. This can be achieved through the fulfilment of various requirements outlined in the IAEA GSR Part 7 (IAEA 2015).

4.2.1.1 Hazard Assessment

Requirement 4 of GSR Part 7 (IAEA 2015) requires that a hazard assessment is conducted to provide a graded approach to a nuclear or radiological emergency. The purpose of the hazard assessment is to identify facilities, activities or sources that would require appropriate response actions in the event of an emergency. These facilities are grouped based on their threat level and their potential consequences from Categories I to V (IAEA 2015). For animal production systems, the categories of primary concern are:

- Category I – Facilities that could give rise to severe deterministic effects off the site
- Category II – Facilities that could give rise to stochastic effects off the site
- Category V – Areas within emergency planning zones and distances of a facility in Category I or II located in another state

These are typically nuclear power plants, research reactors and nuclear-powered vessels.[1] A severe accident at Category I or Category II facilities can result in the distribution of radioactivity over a wide geographical area, leading to contamination of the environment and subsequent contamination of the food chain. For example, the Chernobyl and Fukushima Daiichi accidents are Category I facilities that gave rise radioactive contamination of the environment and food. Hazard assessments should be conducted periodically and bring together information at a national, regional, local and, where appropriate, international level. The results of hazard assessment should be coordinated and shared at a national level with representatives of all organisations that have a role in response to a nuclear or radiological emergency. This is to ensure that all governmental bodies and organisations, including those responsible for agriculture and food production, are in engaged in the hazard analysis.

---

[1] Category III facilities are those that would not warrant actions off-site, for example, industrial irradiation facilities or hospitals.

Category IV are activities or acts that are at an unspecified location, for example, the transport of nuclear or radioactive material.

4.2.1.2 Development, Justification and Optimisation of a Protection Strategy

A protection strategy is developed, justified and optimised based on the hazards identified and on the potential consequences of a nuclear or radiological emergency. Optimisation of the protection strategy can be assisted with the setting of generic criteria. The generic criteria are typically expressed in terms of the dose to humans that would be received if no actions were taken (projected dose) or dose that has been received. The generic criteria are within a range of 20–100 mSv (IAEA 2015) and are set at these levels to avoid the occurrence of severe health effects due to radiation exposure and to reduce the risk of stochastic effects. If the generic criteria are exceeded, protective actions and other response actions are implemented. Table 4.1 outlines the generic criteria for protective actions and other response

Table 4.1 Generic criteria for protective actions and other response actions for food, milk and drinking water to reduce the risk of stochastic effects through the ingestion of contaminated food, milk or drinking water (IAEA 2015)

<table>
<tr><th colspan="3">Generic criteria</th></tr>
<tr><td colspan="3">Urgent protective actions:</td></tr>
<tr><td>Effective dose</td><td>100 mSv in the first 7 days</td><td rowspan="2">Restrictions on food, milk and drinking water and restrictions on the food chain and water supply</td></tr>
<tr><td>Equivalent dose in foetus</td><td>100 mSv in the first 7 days</td></tr>
<tr><td colspan="3">Early protective actions:</td></tr>
<tr><td>Effective dose</td><td>100 mSv in the first year</td><td rowspan="2">Restrictions on food, milk and drinking water and restrictions on the food chain and water supply</td></tr>
<tr><td>Equivalent dose in foetus</td><td>100 mSv in the first year</td></tr>
<tr><td colspan="3">Protective actions:</td></tr>
<tr><td>Effective dose</td><td>10 mSv in the first year from ingestion of food, milk and drinking water</td><td rowspan="2">Restrict consumption, distribution and sale of non-essential food, milk drinking water and water and other commodities including animal feed. Restrict the use and distribution of other commodities. Replace essential food, milk and drinking water as soon as possible or relocate the people affected if replacements are not available</td></tr>
<tr><td>Equivalent dose in foetus</td><td>10 mSv for the full period of in-utero development from ingestion of food, milk and drinking water</td></tr>
<tr><td colspan="3">Response actions to restrict international trade:</td></tr>
<tr><td>Effective dose</td><td>1 mSv per year</td><td rowspan="2">Restrict non-essential international trade of food and other commodities such as animal feed</td></tr>
<tr><td>Equivalent dose in foetus</td><td>1 mSv for the full period of in-utero development</td></tr>
</table>

actions related to food, milk, drinking water and nonfood commodities such as animal feed in an emergency to reduce the risk of stochastic effects.

Generic criteria are based on doses that need to be determined in the preparedness phase taking into account a large number of factors (IAEA 2015). The generic criteria can contain considerable uncertainties; therefore, they cannot be used directly in emergency response where urgent actions are required. Instead a set of operational criteria are derived, in advance, from the generic criteria that can be used directly in an emergency to allow the effective implementation of protective actions including food milk and drinking water restrictions and their associated arrangements. The operational criteria are:

1. The observables at the scene of the nuclear or radiological emergency: Observables can include an unshielded, damaged or potentially damaged source; a major spill from a potentially damaged source; a fire, explosion or fumes from a dangerous source; an earthquake or a suspected radiological dispersal device.
2. Emergency Action Levels (EALs): These are specific, predetermined and observable criteria based on abnormal facility conditions. For Category I and II sites, certain EALs will lead to the declaration of a general emergency, with off-site consequences.
3. Operational Intervention Levels (OILs). OILs are operational criteria that allow the prompt implementation of protective actions and other response actions on the basis of monitoring results that are readily available during a nuclear or radiological emergency.

The relationship between generic criteria and operational criteria are outlined in Fig. 4.2.

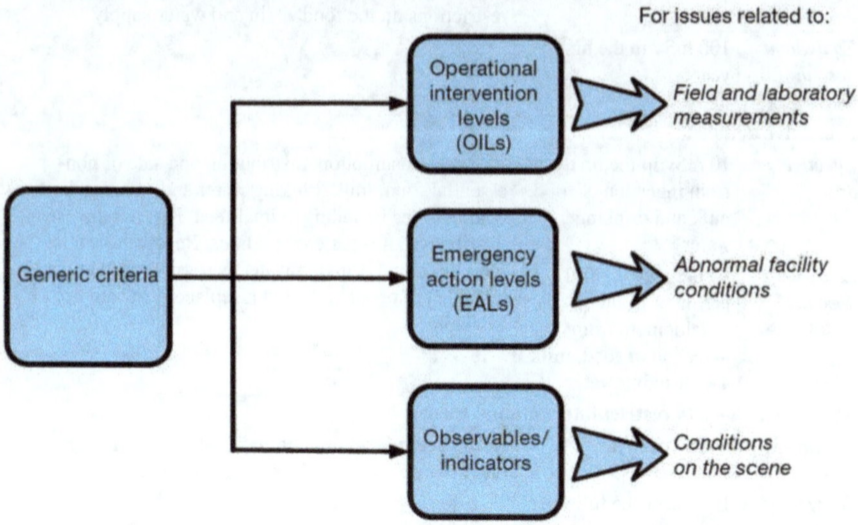

Fig. 4.2 The system of generic criteria and operational criteria

Table 4.2 Codex guideline levels for radionuclides in foods with contamination following a nuclear or radiological emergency for use in international trade (CODEX STAN 2006)

Product name	Representative radionuclides	Guideline level (Bq/kg, fw)
Infant foods	^{238}Pu, ^{239}Pu, ^{240}Pu, ^{241}Am	1
	^{90}Sr, ^{106}Ru, ^{129}I, ^{131}I, ^{235}U	100
	^{35}S, ^{60}Co, ^{89}Sr, ^{103}Ru, ^{134}Cs, ^{137}Cs, ^{144}Ce, ^{192}Ir	1000
	^{3}H, ^{14}C, ^{99}Tc	1000
Foods other than infant foods	^{238}Pu, ^{239}Pu, ^{240}Pu, ^{241}Am	10
	^{90}Sr, ^{106}Ru, ^{129}I, ^{131}I, ^{235}U	100
	^{35}S, ^{60}Co, ^{89}Sr, ^{103}Ru, ^{134}Cs, ^{137}Cs, ^{144}Ce, ^{192}Ir	1000
	^{3}H, ^{14}C, ^{99}Tc	10,000

4.2.1.3 International Trade of Food Following a Nuclear or Radiological Emergency

The trade of food internationally following a nuclear or radiological emergency is governed by the Joint FAO/WHO Codex Alimentarius Commission Guidelines for radionuclides in food (CODEX STAN 2006). Similar to the generic criteria for the restriction of food traded internationally outlined in Table 4.1, the guideline levels are based on a reference level of 1 mSv per year. Assuming 10% of the diet consumed is from imported food, guideline values have been determined for 20 radionuclides for infant foods and other foods other than infant foods. The 20 radionuclides have been divided into four groups based on their radiotoxicity and are outlined in Table 4.2. If food traded internationally are below the guideline levels, then they are deemed safe for human consumption. As these values are only guideline levels, if they are exceeded, national governments will need to determine whether these foods can be traded and consumed within their jurisdiction.

4.2.1.4 OILs for Triggering Food, Milk and Drinking Water Restrictions

The IAEA have derived default OILs for use in a nuclear or radiological emergency based on generic criteria (IAEA 2011). Default OIL values need to be established in the preparedness phase in order to make decisions quickly in the urgent and early phases of an emergency when information is limited.

In the early phase of an emergency, surface contamination measurements are relatively easy to obtain using field survey instruments. OIL 1, OIL 2 and OIL 3 are measurements of ground contamination calling for urgent protective actions, early protective actions and restrictions to be implemented to keep the dose to any person below the generic criteria (for examples of generic criteria, see Table 4.1). This includes the implementation of the appropriate restrictions on food, milk and

Table 4.3 Default OILs for deposition (IAEA 2011)

OIL	OIL value	Protective action for food restrictions if exceeded
OIL 1	Gamma 1000 μSv/h at 1 m from a surface or a source 2000 count(s) direct beta surface contamination measurement 50 count(s) direct alpha surface contamination measurement	Stop consumption of local produce, rainwater and milk from animals grazing in the area
OIL 2	Gamma 100 μSv/h at 1 m from a surface or a source 200 count(s) direct beta surface contamination measurement 10 count(s) direct alpha surface contamination measurement	Stop consumption of local produce, rainwater and milk from animals grazing in the area until they have been screened and contamination levels have been assessed using OIL 5 and OIL 6
OIL 3	Gamma 1 μSv/h at 1 m from a surface or a source 20 count(s) direct beta surface contamination measurement 2 count(s) direct alpha surface contamination measurement	Stop consumption of non-essential local produce, rainwater and milk from animals grazing in the area until it has been screened and contamination levels have been assessed using OIL 5 and OIL 6 Screen local produce, rainwater and milk from animals grazing in the area out to at least ten times the distance to which OIL 3 is exceeded and assesses samples using OIL 5 and OIL 6 Consider providing iodine thyroid blocking for fresh fission products and for iodine contamination if replacement for essential local produce or milk is not immediately available Estimate the dose of those who may have consumed food, milk or rainwater from the area where restrictions were implemented to determine if medical screening is warranted

drinking water. Table 4.3 outlines the default OILs for ground/surface contamination and the response action for food, milk and drinking water if the OIL is exceeded.

If ground/surface contamination measurements indicate the exceedance of generic criteria, food, milk and drinking water, restrictions may be put in place. Further analysis will be required to confirm or lift these restrictions. This requires the analysis of food, milk and drinking water samples. OIL 5 is a screening of potentially contaminated foodstuffs for gross alpha and beta activity. If the gross alpha and beta screening levels are below the OIL 5 values, then the foodstuff is safe to consume in the emergency phase. If the screening level is exceeded, then additional analysis is required to determine the radionuclide-specific concentrations in the food, milk or drinking water; this analysis is based on the use of OIL 6. The collection and analysis of food, milk and drinking water sample analysis of specific radionuclides and comparison with their corresponding OIL 6 values are very time-consuming and complex. Comprehensive activity concentrations in

Table 4.4 Default OILS for contamination of food milk and drinking water (IAEA 2011)

OIL	OIL value	Response action if exceeded
OIL 5	Gross beta, 100 Bq/kg Or Gross alpha, 5 Bq/kg	Assess using OIL 6
OIL 6	$\sum_i \frac{C_{f,i}}{\text{OIL6}_i} > 1$ Where $C_{f,i}$ is the concentration of radionuclide I in the food, milk or water and OIL 6_i is the radionuclide specific OIL for radionuclide *i*	Stop consumption of non-essential food, milk or water and conduct an assessment based on realistic consumption rates. Replace essential food, milk and water promptly, or relocate people if replacement of food, milk and water is not possible For fission products (e.g. containing iodine) and iodine contamination, consider providing iodine thyroid blocking if replacement of essential food, milk or water is not immediately possible Estimate the dose of those who may have consumed food, milk or rainwater from the area where restrictions were implemented to determine if medical screening is warranted
For an emergency at a light water reactor (IAEA 2013a)		
OIL 7	1000 Bq/kg of I-131 Or 200 Bq/kg of Cs-137	Within days: Stop the consumption, distribution and sale of the affected food, milk or drinking water. If the food, milk or drinking water is essential, replace it Within weeks: Estimate the dose from all exposure pathways for those who may have consumed food, milk or drinking water with activity concentrations greater than OIL 7 to determine if medical screening is warranted

food, milk and drinking water may not be readily available in the timeframes required for effective decision-making in the early stages of an emergency. Therefore, the IAEA has defined an additional OIL 7 but for light water reactor emergencies only (IAEA 2013a) (Table 4.3). The OIL 7 values are defined through ^{131}I and ^{137}Cs as marker radionuclides (but they consider all other radionuclides that are likely to be discharged as a result of an emergency at a light water reactor).

Table 4.4 outlines the default OILs for food milk and water along with the response action if the OIL is exceeded.

Restrictions on food, milk and drinking water can be implemented based on generic criteria or OILs only if they are non-essential and there are alternative sources of food, milk or drinking water available. These restrictions cannot be implemented if they would result in severe malnutrition, dehydration or other severe health impacts (IAEA 2015).

For nonfood commodities, for example, animal feed response actions such as restrictions on its use or trade can be developed using OIL_C values. Methods for the derivation of OIL_C values are outlined in IAEA GSG-11 (IAEA 2018a).

Table 4.5 Suggested sizes for emergency zones and distances for light water reactors (IAEA 2013a)

	Suggested maximum radius (km)	
Emergency zones and distances	≥1000 MW(th)	100–1000 MW(th)
Precautionary action zone (PAZ)	3–5	
Urgent protective action planning zone (UPZ)	15–30	
Extended planning distance (EPD)	100	50
Ingestion and commodities planning distance (ICPD)	300	100

4.2.1.5 Emergency Planning Zones and Emergency Planning Distances

In accordance with the development of a protection strategy as outlined in IAEA's GSR Part 7 (IAEA 2015), arrangements need to be made in the preparedness stage to ensure effective decision-making in the taking of urgent protective actions, early protective actions and other response actions. Given the limitations on the information available in the urgent and early phases of an emergency, the response actions are assisted through the establishment of specific off-site emergency planning zones and emergency planning distances (IAEA 2007a). These emergency planning zones and distances are applicable to facilities in Emergency Preparedness Categories I and II and in areas in Emergency Preparedness Category V.

The emergency planning zones and distances include a precautionary action zone (PAZ), an urgent protective action planning zone (UPZ), an extended planning distance (EPD) and an ingestion and commodities planning distance (ICPD). These zones and distances range from a few up to hundreds of kilometres and are contiguous across country borders. Table 4.5 outlines the suggested sizes for the emergency planning zones and emergency planning distances for light water reactors, based on their power levels, but the actual boundaries of these need to be defined by local conditions and landmarks (e.g. roads and rivers) so that they are easily identified during an emergency. An example of these zones and distances for light water reactors can be seen in Fig. 4.3 (IAEA 2013a).

4.2.2 Emergency Exposure Situation

A nuclear or radiological emergency can be declared as a result of an actual or potential release of radioactivity.

Once a nuclear or radiological emergency has been declared, prompt action is required during the emergency exposure situation. The emergency exposure situation can be divided into three phases as outlined in Fig. 4.1. The timeline of these phases is dependent on the nature and scale of the nuclear or radiological emergency. The sequence of protective actions as a result of a nuclear or radiological emergency is outlined in Fig. 4.4.

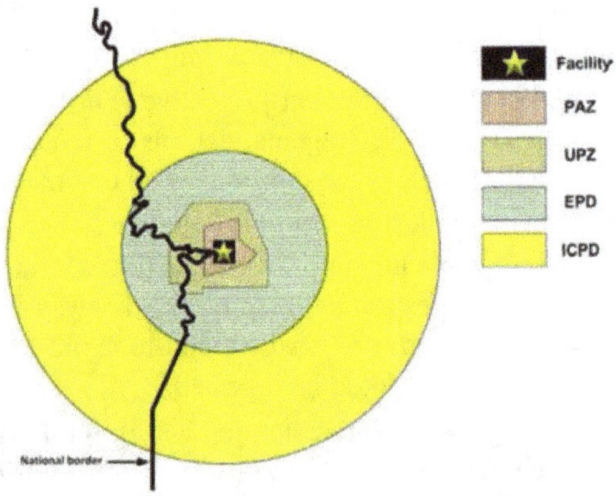

Fig. 4.3 Emergency planning zones and emergency planning distances (IAEA 2013a)

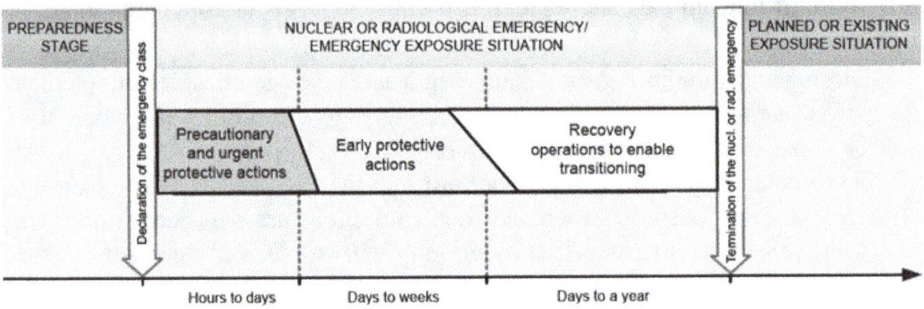

Fig. 4.4 Temporal sequence of various types of protective actions and recovery options for a nuclear or radiological emergency (IAEA 2018a)

4.2.2.1 The Urgent Response Phase

The urgent response phase is the period in which actions must be taken within hours or days to be effective; these are the precautionary and urgent protective actions that have been predetermined in the preparedness phase and are based on observables and conditions at a facility (e.g. the declaration of a general emergency).

Precautionary urgent protective actions are implemented before or shortly after a release of radioactive material to avoid severe deterministic effects. For Category I facilities, the precautionary urgent protective actions include the consumption of an ITB agent, the safe evacuation of the PAZ beyond the UPZ and food, milk and drinking water restrictions. These precautionary urgent protective actions should take place within an hour of the declaration of a general emergency (IAEA 2013a).

Urgent protective actions need to be implemented within hours or days of the declaration of an emergency to maximise their effectiveness. These actions include evacuation, short-term sheltering, actions to reduce inadvertent ingestion, decontamination of individuals and protection of the food and water supplies, restrictions on significantly contaminated food and water supplies and the provision of instructions to protect agricultural products. These urgent protective actions are implemented within the predetermined emergency planning zones and distances.

Within the UPZ, urgent protective actions can include sheltering or evacuation, administering of ITB agents, actions to reduce inadvertent ingestion and instructions to the public not to consume food that may have been directly contaminated or to consume milk from animals that may graze on contaminated ground.

The principle urgent protective action within the EPD is to take actions to reduce inadvertent ingestion by keeping hands away from the mouth, not to drink, eat or smoke until hands are washed, and to avoid activities that could result in the creation of dust that could be ingested.

The urgent protective actions within the ICPD are to place grazing animals on protected feed if feasible, to protect food and drinking water sources and to stop the consumption and distribution of non-essential local produce, wild-grown produce, milk from grazing animals and animal feed until the levels of contamination have been assessed.

Environmental monitoring should also begin as soon as practicable to implement the appropriate restrictions on food and drinking water from rainwater where they may be contaminated to levels requiring restrictions. In practice, it may only be feasible to conduct ground/surface monitoring in the PAZ and UPZ to determine whether OIL 3 has been exceeded and food restrictions are required. Further and more comprehensive environmental monitoring will be required during the subsequent phases of the emergency.

Following the declaration of an emergency, specific urgent protective actions can be implemented before and shortly after the release of radioactivity to the environment to reduce the risk of contamination of animals. Such actions include (Nisbet et al. 2015):

- Short-term sheltering of animals
- Provision of clean feed
- Covering of harvested fodder
- Closure of air intake valves at food processing plants

These urgent protective actions are applicable for areas in threat Categories I, II and V.

4.2.2.2 The Early Response Phase

At the early response phase, the radiological situation has been sufficiently characterised to enable the implementation of actions that are effective within days or weeks; these are the early protective actions.

Early protective actions are those pre-established in the preparedness phase and are based on operational criteria, such as OILs, until more detailed characterisation of radioactivity in the environment and laboratory analysis of food, milk and water samples are conducted in the transition phase.

The environmental monitoring, sampling and laboratory analysis can be used to start adjusting the initial protective actions implemented in the urgent response phase to confirm the adequacy of the controls in place, to provide for additional protective actions or to remove restrictions. This could lead to:

- Longer-term restrictions on food, milk and drinking water
- Relocation of people if they are living in areas where essential food and drinking water is contaminated and replacements cannot be provided
- Actions to prevent contaminated food and animal feed from entering the food chain

There may also be a need to revise the OIL values and to extend monitoring and assessment beyond the initial emergency planning zones and distances to take into account the conditions during the emergency. This could lead to additional restrictions or the lifting of restrictions on food, milk and drinking water in certain areas.

Consideration also needs to be given to the protection of international trade and commercial interests, and restrictions can be placed on food and commodities from affected areas until it has been verified that they do not exceed internationally agreed criteria for trade (IAEA 2013b).

The early response phase is the time where other agricultural countermeasures can begin to be implemented in order to protect the food chain and to avert dose over longer time periods. In addition to the early protective actions listed above, the other protective actions considered most effective for animal production systems in the early phase are (Nisbet et al. 2015):

- Slaughtering of animals or dairy livestock shortly after deposition
- Restrictions on the gathering of wild foods, hunting and fishing
- Suppression of lactation before slaughter to avoid the production of contaminated milk

4.2.2.3 The Transition Phase

The transition phase commences once the radioactive source is under control, the situation is stable and the radiological situation is well understood. Once this occurs there is a progression to the point at which the emergency can be terminated through the reduction of long-term exposures and the improvement of living conditions in the affected areas (IAEA 2018a).

At this phase of the emergency the actions implemented are, in a large part, remedial or recovery actions as the more disruptive protective actions have been implemented in the urgent and early response phases. Furthermore, the actions in the transition phase are not driven by urgency and can be justified and optimised through consultation with interested parties, whereas in the earlier phases of an emergency, consultation with interested parties is limited.

A number of aspects need to be considered at the preparedness phase when establishing arrangements for the transition phase. Three key elements to be considered for animal production systems are:

- The lifting or adapting of protective actions
- Radioactive waste management
- Dealing with non-radiological affects

The protective actions that were implemented in the urgent and early response phases are based on operational criteria that were predetermined in the emergency preparedness phase and on the limited environmental monitoring that is conducted in the early response phase.

OILs can be used to consider which specific protective actions can be lifted or adapted. For example, restrictions on food, milk and drinking water in the urgent and early response phases were based on EALs and OIL3. OIL 5, OIL 6 and/or OIL 7 can be used to adjust any restrictions imposed. In the transition phase, a comprehensive sampling and monitoring programme is carried out to determine the levels of radioactivity in the environment and in food, milk and drinking water. This detailed radiological characterisation can be used to determine the dose in the future after protective actions have been lifted, i.e. the residual dose. The residual dose can be determined once the exposure pathways have been characterised and the urgent and early protective actions are known.

The final decision on the adapting or lifting protective actions are based on these residual dose assessments. In order to terminate an emergency, the residual dose should be in the order of 20 mSv effective dose in a year (IAEA 2015). In the transition phase, after more comprehensive sampling and monitoring of food, milk and drinking water, the actual dose from ingestion can be calculated, and its contribution to the residual dose can be estimated to determine whether this protective action can be adapted or lifted (IAEA 2018a).

The lifting or adapting of protective actions may also be possible through the implementation of decontamination and dose reduction techniques. In animal production systems, the techniques that can be used in the transition phase for dose reduction are (Nisbet et al. 2015):

- Selective grazing whereby animals are restricted from grazing on highly contaminated land and moved to pastures with lower contamination
- The addition of additives to animal feed to inhibit the uptake of radionuclides
- Decontamination or processing of milk to reduce the radioactivity levels
- Live monitoring of animals to determine whether clean feeding or the addition of additives to feed can be implemented before slaughter to reduce levels of significant contamination

4.2.2.4 Radioactive Waste Management

The management of radioactive waste increases in importance in the transition phase of an emergency response as, earlier in an emergency, the focus is primarily on implementing protective actions. Large-scale nuclear or radiological emergencies can generate large volumes of radioactive waste capable of overwhelming national capabilities for radioactive waste management and delaying the termination of an emergency. The waste generated during a nuclear or radiological emergency can be as a result of the emergency situation or could arise from the protective actions or other response actions implemented during the emergency (IAEA 1987, 2013b).

Before the disposal of any waste arising from a nuclear or radiological emergency, it needs to be identified, characterised and categorised taking into account the various radiological and non-radiological (chemical, biological, physical and mechanical) aspects of the waste. This should be based on regulations on radioactive waste management that should be developed in the preparedness phase. Methodologies also need to be developed in advance for the identification of appropriate storage options and sites and the predisposal management of radioactive waste through segregation, packing, transport and storage. Arrangements should also be made to minimise the amount of waste declared as radioactive waste through the introduction of clearance levels for waste materials or through the reuse or recycling of the waste.

Consideration should also be given to obtain international assistance in waste management.

In animal production systems, the management of animal remains also needs to be given special consideration. For animal production systems, management options need to be identified for the disposal of animal carcasses. Workers handling the animal carcasses need to be trained in basic radiation protection principles, and they need to be provided with the appropriate equipment to ensure their exposure to radioactivity is kept to a minimum (IAEA 2013b).

The disposal options that can be considered in the transition phase include (Nisbet et al. 2015):

- The biological treatment of contaminated milk through aerobic and anaerobic digestion
- The disposal of contaminated milk to sea
- The burial or burning of animal carcasses following slaughter
- Disposal of contaminated food to landfill with an option of incineration beforehand to reduce the volume being disposed
- Landspreading of contaminated milk and/or contaminated slurry
- Rendering of animal carcasses to reduce volumes before disposal

4.2.2.5 Dealing with Non-radiological Consequences

In the early stages of emergency response, the radiological issues typically outweigh non-radiological consequences, but in the transition phase, as doses tend to decrease with the effective implementation of protective and recovery actions, non-radiological factors become increasingly important. These non-radiological consequences include psychosocial, economic and political factors and require the active participation of the public and other interested parties in the transition phase. This can include the psychosocial impact of farm and veterinary workers in areas affected by radioactive contamination. For example, farmers concern about growing or selling produce (Takebayahi et al. 2017).

A nuclear or radiological emergency and the protective actions implemented in the emergency response phase can have a detrimental impact on the economy, trade and people's livelihood. Therefore, compensation for the damage caused by nuclear or radiological emergencies may be required in these instances. This was demonstrated in the United Kingdom in the wake of the Chernobyl accident in 1986 where farmers where compensated for market losses incurred on sheep sold at auction (Kerr and Mooney 1988; IAEA 2018a).

4.2.3 The Termination of a Nuclear or Radiological Emergency

The termination of a nuclear or radiological emergency is based on a formal decision that is made public and is made in consultation with interested parties. The termination of the emergency takes into consideration both radiological and non-radiological consequences and can be implemented at different times and in different geographical areas depending on the nature and scale of the emergency (IAEA 2015).

A nuclear or radiological emergency can only be terminated once a number of general and specific prerequisites have been met. The source of the nuclear or radiological emergency should be under control, the future development of the situation is well understood and no further significant releases or exposures should be expected. All of the urgent and early protective actions should be implemented, with the possibility that some may already be lifted or adapted, and the radiological situation should be well characterised with doses assessed for the affected populations. This includes the dose ingested through the consumption of food from animal production systems. The radiological situation should be assessed against the appropriate reference levels, generic criteria and operational criteria to determine whether the residual dose of the affected population is at or below approximately 20 mSv per year (IAEA 2018a).

Once all the prerequisites for the termination of an emergency have been met, the emergency exposure situation ends, and the end of the emergency can be declared.

4.2.4 *Planned or Existing Exposure Situation*

Once the emergency has been terminated the situation moves to either a planned or existing exposure situation (Fig. 4.1).

Nuclear or radiological emergencies that do not result in a significant release of radioactivity into the environment and do not result in long-term exposure of individuals due to residual radioactive material can transition to a planned exposure situation. In these circumstances, these situations are not expected to result in an exposure situation that differs from one that existed prior to the emergency (IAEA 2018a).

An emergency that has resulted in a significant release of radioactive material to the environment, typically a nuclear emergency, will result in exposure during the emergency and in the long term due to residual radioactivity in the environment. For these situations, once the end of an emergency has been declared, the situation transitions to an existing exposure situation (IAEA 1987, 2013b, 2018a).

The IAEA requirements and guidance for planned and existing exposure situations are governed by additional IAEA safety standards series publications and include but not limited:

- General Safety Requirements No. GSR Part 3 – Radiation Protection and Safety of Radiation Sources: International Basic Safety Standards (IAEA 2013b)
- General Safety Guide No. GSG-8 – Radiation Protection of the Public and the Environment (IAEA 2018b)
- Safety Guide No. WSG-3.1 – Remediation Process for Areas Affected by Past Activities and Accidents (IAEA 2007b)

4.2.4.1 Restrictions on Food, Milk and Drinking Water After the Termination of an Emergency

Once the end of an emergency has been declared, any restrictions implemented on food, milk or drinking water are no longer governed by the requirements for emergency exposure situations (IAEA 2016). Instead, for existing exposure situations, the framework is governed by the WHO Guidelines for Drinking-Water Quality (WHO 2011) and the IAEA GSR Part 3 (IAEA 2013c). The WHO Guidelines for drinking water quality sets a reference level of 0.1 mSv per year for consumption of drinking water from all sources of radioactivity. Requirement 51 of GSR Part 3 requires regulatory bodies to establish reference levels for exposure due to food, feed and drinking water based on a dose that doesn't exceed a value of about 1 mSv per year.

For food used in international trade, the Codex Alimentarius guidelines outlined above still apply in an existing exposure situation (CODEX STAN 2006).

Following any nuclear or radiological emergency, it is important that arrangements remain in place to reassure the public and interested parties (such as trading partners) that the food meets international standards. This can be achieved through a testing and certification system that can verify that food products are safe and do not exceed the reference levels and internationally agreed criteria for trade (IAEA 2013a).

References

CODEX STAN. (2006). Joint FAO/WHO food standards programme, Codex Alimentarius Commission, "Codex General Standard for Contaminants and Toxins in Foods, Schedule 1 – Radionuclides, CODEX STAN 193–1995. Rome: CAC.

IAEA. (1987). *Convention on early notification of a nuclear accident and convention on assistance in the case of a nuclear accident or radiological emergency* (Legal series no. 14). Vienna: IAEA.

IAEA. (2007a). *Arrangements for preparedness for a nuclear or radiological emergency* (IAEA safety standards series no. GS-G-2.1). Vienna: IAEA.

IAEA. (2007b). *Remediation process for areas affected by past activities and accidents* (IAEA safety standards series no. WS-G-3.1). Vienna: IAEA.

IAEA. (2011). *Criteria for use in preparedness and response for a nuclear or radiological emergency* (IAEA safety standards series no. GSG-2). Vienna: IAEA.

IAEA. (2013a). *Actions to protect the public in an emergency due to severe conditions at a light water reactor* (EPR-NPP public protective actions). Vienna: IAEA.

IAEA. (2013b). *Radiation protection and safety of radiation sources: International basic safety standards* (IAEA safety standards series no. GSR part 3). Vienna: IAEA.

IAEA. (2015). *Preparedness and response for a nuclear or radiological emergency* (IAEA safety standards series no. GSR part 7). Vienna: IAEA.

IAEA. (2016). *Criteria for radionuclide activity concentrations for food and drinking water*. Vienna: IAEA.

IAEA. (2018a). *Arrangements for the termination of a nuclear or radiological emergency* (General safety guide no. GSG-11). Vienna: IAEA.

IAEA. (2018b). *Radiation protection of the public and the environment* (IAEA safety standards series no. GSG-8). Vienna: IAEA.

Kerr, W., & Mooney, S. (1988). A system disrupted – The grazing economy of North Wales in the wake of Chernobyl. *Agricultural Systems, 28*(1), 13–27.

Nisbet, A., Watson, S., & Public Health England. Centre for Radiation, Chemical and Environmental Hazards. (2015). *UK recovery handbooks for radiation incidents*. Chilton: PHE.

Takebayahi, Y., Lyamzina, Y., & Suzuki, Y. (2017). Risk perception and anxiety regarding radiation after the 2011 Fukushima nuclear power plant accident: A systematic qualitative review. *International Journal of Environmental Research and Public Health, 14*(11), 1306.

WHO. (2011). *Guidelines for drinking-water quality – 4th edition*. Geneva: WHO.

5

Radionuclides: Contaminants in Animals and Animal Products

Brenda Howard

This chapter briefly describes the NREs which released large amounts of radionuclides that had the potential to cause significant contamination of animals and animal products. It then describes the key environmental and metabolic pathways of animals and animal product contamination. The different methods used to quantify the transfer of radionuclides between relevant environmental pathways are also described. Radionuclide-specific information is provided in subsequent sections. Observed effects on agricultural and game animals after two NREs are also described.

5.1 Major Nuclear or Radiological Emergencies Causing Animal and Animal Product Contamination

There have been a range of different NREs that have contaminated animal and animal products. Animal products have been contaminated after all of the four largest NREs that have occurred from nuclear reactors or waste storage facilities. Estimated radionuclide releases from these four sources are listed in Table 5.1. Most of the radionuclides listed in Table 5.1 may be important contributors to internal exposure to humans via animal products after a NRE.

Although many different radionuclides can be released following a NRE, some are short-lived, and others do not readily transfer into food. Additional radionuclides, not listed above, of potential relevance for animal products after NREs include ^{3}H, ^{14}C, ^{35}S, ^{60}Co, ^{95}Nb, ^{99}Tc, ^{103}Ru, ^{106}Ru, ^{110}Ag, ^{129}I, ^{132}Te, ^{192}Ir, ^{235}U and ^{241}Am. The relative importance of these different radionuclides varies depending on the magnitude of the release and on environmental and agricultural husbandry

B. Howard (✉)
School of Biosciences, Nottingham University, Nottingham, UK

Table 5.1 Estimated releases of selected radioisotopes for the four largest NREs which led to animal product contamination

Radioactive atmospheric releases (TBq)				
Isotopes	Kyshtym	Windscale	Chernobyl	Fukushima Daiichi
Reference source	Akleyev et al. (2017)	Garland and Wakeford (2007)	UNSCEAR (2011)	IAEA (2015)
^{131}I		1800	1,760,000	100,000–400,000
^{137}Cs	260	180	~85,000	7000–20,000
^{134}Cs		12	~47,000	8300–50,000
^{210}Po		42		
^{90}Sr	4000	0.75	10,000	3.3–140
Pu isotopes	1.5	0.02	46[a] and 2600[b]	0.0034–0.025[a] and 0.0003–1.2[b]
^{95}Zr	18,400	16	84,000	17
^{144}Ce and ^{141}Ce	48,700	13	134,000	29
^{106}Ru	2700	3	>73,000	0.002

[a]Pu alpha
[b] ^{241}Pu

characteristics. For animals and animal products, it also depends heavily on the extent to which the radioisotopes are accumulated by animal tissues – this issue is addressed in Sect. 5.4.3.

Examples of the features controlling the contamination of animal products and their consequences are given in this chapter based on information acquired after each of the four NREs.

5.2 Key Environmental Processes Controlling Animal Product Contamination

There are a large number of different environmental factors which affect the extent to which radionuclides, such as those listed in Table 5.1, will accumulate in animals and animal products in the human food chain. Some factors are more important in the emergency phase after a NRE whilst others are more relevant in the transition to recovery phases.

They include:

- Interception on, and loss from, plant surfaces
- Chemical form
- Soil fixation processes
- Rates of plant uptake
- Diet of food-producing animals
- Absorption rates in the gut of animals

- Transfer rates to tissues (including milk)
- Dynamic changes with time in tissue contamination
- Diet and habits of humans

Some of these processes are highly dependent on which radionuclides have been released (such as soil fixation and gut absorption), whereas others are not (such as interception and human dietary preferences).

There are definable situations where there is substantial transfer of radionuclides into food products caused by particular features of the release or the contaminated system. In such situations, the feature is considered to be radioecologically sensitive to that radionuclide (Howard 2000). A typical example is the presence of certain soil types which fail to permanently fix radiocaesium ions to soil particles, thereby allowing continued transfer into the soil solution and subsequent uptake by plants and then animals (Fig. 5.1).

Milk and meat products can become contaminated rapidly, especially if radionuclides are released to the atmosphere. Radionuclides in milk can be a major source of internal dose via the human food chain soon after a release. Radioiodine (especially ^{131}I), radiocaesium (^{134}Cs and ^{137}Cs) and ^{90}Sr are often key components of ingestion dose via animal products, potentially over decades for ^{137}Cs and ^{90}Sr. The radioactive contamination of animals and animal products impacts not only on farmers and consumers but also on agricultural and regulatory ministries and the

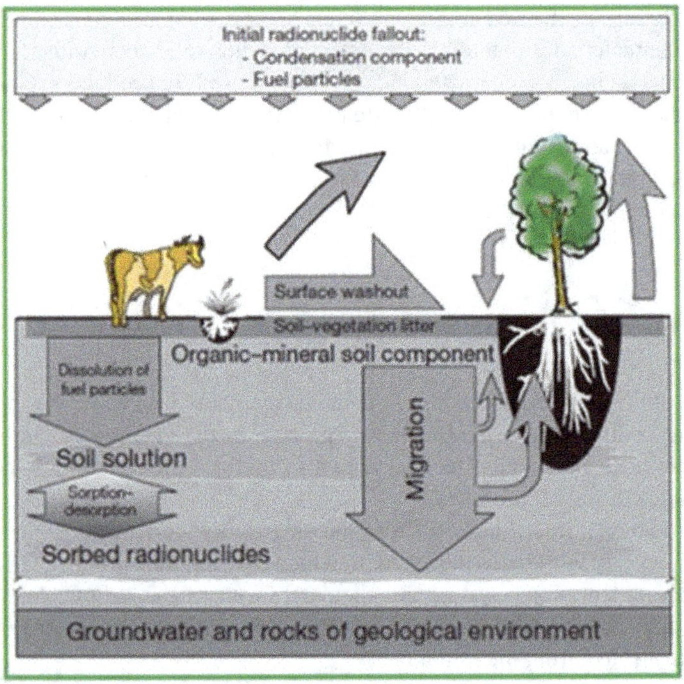

Fig. 5.1 Routes of radionuclide transfer in the environment (IAEA 2006a)

food industry. Professional groups that may be involved in the response to a NRE need to be informed about how animal products become contaminated and what controls the extent to which major radionuclides will be retained in, or lost from, animal tissues.

There are a number of different routes through which agricultural, free-ranging domesticated animals and game animals may become contaminated with radionuclides released from NREs. The key routes of contamination are:

- Inhalation into the lung of gaseous radionuclides or particulates present in the atmosphere, or of resuspended contaminated material such as windblown soil particles. Such pathways are only relevant for emergency stages after a NRE when radionuclides may be present in the air.
- Direct uptake of radionuclides in volatile, gaseous forms via plant stomata.
- Direct deposition of radionuclides onto external surfaces of plants (such as leaves, bark, grain and other edible parts) and animals (such as fur, feathers, skin).
- Ingestion of plants, fungi and soil contaminated with radionuclides by animals.
- Ingestion of contaminated water from sources such as water butts, surfaces of plants, puddles and streams by animals.

The relative importance of the above routes of contamination of animal products in the human food chain depends on the environmental pathways. The importance of these pathways depends on many factors such as the time of year that the NRE happened, the radionuclides released and the prevailing animal production or harvesting practices in affected areas.

Other characteristics that affect the extent of radionuclide contamination of animal products include the characteristics of the land used for production (such as the soil type and plant uptake rates), the extent of gastrointestinal absorption, the metabolic fate in the animal and the rate of loss from tissues (principally in urine, faeces and milk). These pathways are described in more detail below, focusing on aspects relating to the human food chain.

5.2.1 Vegetation Interception

The interception and retention of radionuclides by plants which are then consumed by grazing or browsing animals is a key process in the emergency phase after a NRE. It provides a fast and effective route for initial transfer of recently deposited radionuclides to animal products.

Once radionuclides are released into the air (or to water), various physical and chemical processes influence the extent to which they are transported and dispersed in the environment. The physical and chemical forms of the radionuclide, and the turbulence of the receiving medium (such as air movements and water flow), play an important role during the initial phase.

Other processes affect the transfer of radionuclides from the air (or the water column) to the receiving surface. Potential deposition mechanisms include:

- Aerosols washed from the atmosphere during precipitation
- Gravitational settling of suspended particulate material in the atmospheric or aquatic releases
- Impaction, whereby suspended particles come into contact with solid objects within an air or water stream
- Chemical sorption and exchange, dependent on both the chemical and physical form of the radionuclide and the interacting surface

Radionuclides interact with solid materials such as soil particles and sediments in many different ways including electrostatic attraction and the formation of chemical bonds. The radionuclide activity concentration per unit mass of solid is affected by the surface area available for adsorption per unit mass or volume and is, therefore, greater for smaller objects. In terrestrial areas, the interception of radionuclides by vegetation occurs for both wet and dry deposition.

Wet deposition occurs when radionuclides in air are washed out by precipitation. Vegetation surfaces retain a fraction of radionuclides deposited with the rain, with the remaining fractions falling onto the ground. The fraction of radionuclides in the air that is initially intercepted is an important quantity in radioecological models because direct deposition can lead to relatively high activity concentrations in pasture grazed by animals, and other feed crops.

Plants with a relatively high biomass per unit area will intercept more radionuclides in wet deposition, associated with a higher interception fraction. Other factors such as the capacity of the canopy to retain water, ionic form of the radionuclide, precipitation amount and intensity, vegetation maturity and leaf area index (LAI – upper-side green leaf area per unit ground surface area) can all influence the extent of interception of wet deposition (IAEA 2009). For example, the interception fraction of ^{137}Cs by grass was reported to decline with increasing intensity of rainfall from 0.1 to 0.2 for low rates of up to 1 mm of rainfall to an order of magnitude lower at higher rates of 11 mm of rainfall (Kinnersley et al. 1997).

Most of the intercepted radionuclides are gradually transferred to the soil and are only temporarily present on the surface of the vegetation. Radionuclide activity concentrations on vegetation may be reduced by various physical processes, including wash-off by rain or irrigation, surface abrasion, leaf bending from wind action, resuspension, tissue senescence, leaf fall, herbivore grazing, growth and evaporation.

Interception and retention of radionuclides on plant surfaces is a critical process in the emergency phase after a NRE. If a NRE occurs before the growing season, the likely transfer of radionuclides to grazing animals will be low, but may still occur if stored feed is not covered or animals are kept outdoors. Conversely, a NRE occurring at the height of the growing season with light rainfall when plant biomass is high and animals are outside grazing pasture may present an immediate problem to responding authorities. After the Chernobyl NRE, dairy cows in affected areas of the USSR were grazing pasture which had sufficient leaf mass in late April and early May to intercept significant amounts of radioiodine and radiocaesium.

Dry deposition is dependent on the characteristics of the intercepting surface, usually quantified using the surface roughness (Heinemann and Vogt 1980), which generally increases as the plant canopy develops. The extent of interception for dry deposition depends on the standing biomass of plants, the chemical form and the particle size of the deposit. Interception is similar for small (up to a few micrometres diameter) particles, but as particle size increases, interception decreases probably because larger particles roll off the plant surface more easily than smaller ones. Furthermore, if vegetation is moist or wet, absorption increases possibly due to an enhanced stickiness. Particles with a diameter up to a few micrometres are relatively more important because larger particles from a radioactive cloud are rapidly depleted. As for wet deposits, the extent of interception of dry deposits depends on many factors including plant yield, particle size, the crop, the chemical form and whether the receiving surface characteristics are wet or dry.

Although relatively minor in comparison to the above routes, stored crops intended as fodder for animals may become contaminated by surface deposits of radionuclides if they are not covered outdoors.

Information is available on how to quantify interception in IAEA documents TECDOC 1616 and TRS 472 (IAEA 2009, 2010).

5.2.2 *Chemical Form of the Released Radionuclides*

The chemical form of the released radionuclides impacts on many different pathways, including the extent of interception, the rate at which radionuclides are released into the soil solution and are then available for plant uptake and the ability of the radionuclide to be absorbed in the animal's GI tract. Examples of the impact of chemical form will be given in the relevant sections below.

5.2.3 *Radionuclide Behaviour in Soils*

Plants take up nutrients and pollutants from the soil solution, so the radionuclide activity concentration in soil solution is a critical determining factor for plant uptake. The activity concentration of radionuclides in soil solution is determined by processes influencing the loss of radionuclides that are adsorbed onto soil components that move into the soil solution usually by competitive ion exchange (quantified as the cation exchange capacity). The concentration and composition of other elements present in the soil are important in determining radionuclide distribution between soil and soil solution. The amount and nature of clay minerals in soils and the concentrations of competitive major cations are often key factors in determining exchange mechanisms in soils of radionuclides, but other factors, such as microbial activity, may also affect radionuclide mobility.

In the emergency and transition phases of a NRE, radionuclide movement into the soil solution may be relatively high, leading to high initial contamination of plants via root uptake. With time the availability of radionuclides in soil solution tends to reduce as radionuclides gradually adsorb to soil components. The rate of reduction varies with radionuclide and soil type.

Vertical migration of radionuclides down the soil column arises from various transport mechanisms including convection, dispersion, diffusion and biological mixing. Radionuclides can also migrate to deeper soil layers at faster rates when there is a high amount of rainfall over a short period of time, especially if there are surface cracks in dry soil or when soils contain a relatively large proportion of sand particles. Soil-dwelling animals can also relocate material both laterally and vertically during the construction of burrows, tunnels and chambers, and the roots of plants can cause a similar effect.

Large-scale lateral migration of radionuclides can also occur in catchments and is often associated with soil erosion or heavy rainfall events such as typhoons. The distribution of radionuclides in sediment or soil layers of the floodplain can be considerably altered by such events.

A high rate of radionuclide vertical migration in soil matter may be beneficial as it will remove radionuclides out of the rooting zone, thereby reducing external doses and plant uptake for surface routing species. However, for many undisturbed soils, most of the deposited radiocaesium is retained in the upper 10 cm layer.

5.2.4 Radionuclide Transfer from Soil to Crops

The uptake of radionuclides, as for other trace elements by plant roots, is a competitive physiological process (IAEA 2010). The processes influencing radionuclide transport from soil to plants vary with both radionuclide and soil type. The fraction of deposited radionuclides taken up by plant roots can differ by orders of magnitude between different elements and between different physico-chemical forms of the same radionuclide. There are also differences in radionuclide uptake between plant species growing on the same soil type.

There will probably be a decrease with time in the activity concentrations of most radionuclides in plants after a short-duration release of radionuclides into the environment due to the gradual fixation by soils (and sediments) discussed above.

After the initial emergency exposure situation of a few months to a year, the dominant processes determining radionuclide movement in farming systems change. The extent to which radionuclides transfer from soil into agricultural products during the later planned or existing exposure situation depends not only on the density of contamination but also on soil type, moisture regime, texture, agrochemical properties and the plant species. The impact of differing radioecological sensitivities of soils is often more important in explaining spatial variation in transfer of radionuclides in agricultural systems. Therefore, identification of radioecologically sensitive areas for animals and animal products is based on both the deposition density of different radionuclides and their mobility within different types of soil.

In terrestrial systems, wind action and rain "splash" on the soil can reintroduce radionuclides to the air where they can be ingested (if deposited on vegetation surfaces) or inhaled by animals. Such resuspension and soil adhesion are influenced by the height and type of the plant canopy as well as weather (wind, rain), soil type and animal trampling. Grazed plants are likely to include radionuclides associated with soil adhered to the plant, as well as being incorporated within the plant itself. For radionuclides with a low transfer from soil to plant, the soil adhered on the surface of pasture grass may be the major source of radionuclide ingested by grazing ruminants. For example, root uptake of plutonium is negligible compared to direct contamination of leaves via adhered soil from rain splash or resuspension, so most ingested plutonium will be associated with adhered soil, especially for pastures with a low plant biomass.

5.2.5 Quantification of Radionuclide Transfer to Plants and Fodder Crops

The transfer from soil to plants is commonly quantified using the concentration ratio (CR) (also called a transfer factor (TF)), which is equal to the plant mass activity concentration (often in Bq/kg dw), divided by soil activity concentration, Bq/kg (dw). Available CR transfer parameter values for a wide range of radionuclides and crops for different soil types are available free in the downloadable TECDOC 1616 (IAEA 2009) and TRS 472 (IAEA 2010).

5.2.6 Intake and Absorption of Radionuclides by Animals

The transfer of radionuclides from plants (and soil) to herbivores occurs mainly by ingestion, although uptake via water can contribute to intake in the emergency phase if water sources have become contaminated after the deposition of radionuclides.

Animal products can be contaminated within a few hours of radionuclide release, mainly by the consumption of contaminated food and, to a lesser extent, water. Contamination through the skin is infrequent and absorption by inhalation is marginal for most radionuclides. The most radioecologically sensitive scenario is that of animals grazing outdoors that are directly consuming contaminated plants which have intercepted radionuclides on their surfaces.

For radionuclides that are not readily taken up by plants, soil adhesion can represent the most important route of intake especially since topsoil tends to be much more contaminated than plant material (IAEA 1994). In some instances, soil ingestion by animals may be deliberate (e.g. to obtain essential minerals), but soil can also be ingested by licking or preening of fur, feathers or offspring (Whicker and Schultz 1982). Radionuclides that are adsorbed to soil matrices may be less bioavailable than when incorporated into plant material for transfer into animal products.

Animals that are housed in pens and barns and given previously stored food (as long as that is protected from fallout) will not be significantly affected although the source of water would need to be identified. Surface water systems can be initially directly contaminated by deposited radionuclides, but dilution in water bodies normally greatly reduces the radionuclide activity concentrations in water.

5.2.7 *Gastrointestinal Absorption*

Absorption of radionuclides from the gastrointestinal tract (GI tract) of animals depends on, amongst other factors, the physico-chemical form of the radionuclide, the composition of the feed and the nutritional status of the animal.

Although absorption can occur through the skin and lungs, oral ingestion of radionuclides in feed, and subsequent absorption through the GI tract, is the major route of entry of radionuclides. The absorbed fraction (F_a) is defined as the fraction of that ingested by animals that is transferred through the GI tract and is a key factor determining the extent of radionuclide contamination of animal tissues and milk. The absorbed fraction depends on many different factors including metabolic status (e.g. age, lactation state, physiological condition), chemical and physical speciation of the radionuclide and the presence of competing ions.

The method of determination of GI tract absorption is important. An apparent absorption is derived from information on the whole-body intake and excretion of the radionuclide. A true absorption value is measured in a metabolic study that involves injection of a tracer which enables determination of endogenous faecal excretion (i.e. direct transfer from blood to the intestine). Endogenous secretion from tissues into the gut occurs for the key radionuclide, radiocaesium, so it is important to distinguish whether reported values refer to an apparent or true absorption value.

Available information on the fractional absorption values for radionuclides in ruminants is available in the TECDOC 1616 and TRS 472 (IAEA 2009, 2010). Fractional absorption values for the most well-studied radionuclide elements are given in Table 5.2. The number of data available on F_a in ruminants for different radionuclides varies, and, therefore, so does the confidence attributable to each

Table 5.2 Range in fractional GI tract absorption values (F_a) for different elements in domestic ruminants

Fractional absorption magnitude	Radionuclide
0.1–1	I, Cl, Na, Cs, P, Se, Ca, Te, Zn, Sr, Fe
0.01–0.1	Ag, Ba, Co, Pb, U
0.001–0.01	Mn, Ru, Cd, Y
0.0001–0.001	Zr, Ce, Pm, Am, Nb
0.00001–0.0001	Pu

Howard et al. (2016a)

Table 5.3 Fractional absorption values for adult humans

Radionuclide	Fractional absorption
H, C, Cs, S, Mo, I	1
Se	0.8
Zn, Tc, Po	0.5
Te, Sr, Ca	0.3
Ba, Ra, Pb	0.2
Co, Fe, Sb	0.1
Ru, Ni, Ag	0.05
U	0.02
Zr, Nb	0.01
Ce, Th, Np, Pu, Am, Cm	0.0005

ICRP (2006)

value. The F_a values vary from almost negligible, in the case of actinides such as plutonium, to 100% for radioiodine (Howard et al. 2009a, 2016a). Data on F_a for iodine, caesium and strontium are considered in more detail in Sect. 6.4.

The compiled ruminant F_a values for radionuclides or stable elements are similar to those reported by the International Commission on Radiological Protection (ICRP) shown in Table 5.3 for humans (and relevant for other monogastric animals such as pigs). Therefore, if ruminant-specific F_a values are not available, those given for humans may be used instead.

After absorption, radionuclides circulate in the blood to different tissues as discussed below.

5.2.8 *Quantification of Radionuclide Transfer to Animal Products*

To quantify the transfer of radionuclides to milk and meat, two types of parameter values are commonly used: transfer coefficients (F_m for milk and F_f for other tissues) and concentration ratios (CR) as follows:

Transfer coefficient (d/kg or d/L)

$$F_m \text{ or } F_f = \frac{\text{Equilibrium activity concentration in food product } (Bq/\text{kg } fw)}{\text{Daily intake of radionuclide } (Bq/\text{d})}$$

Concentration ratio

$$CR = \frac{\text{Equilibrium activity concentration in food product } (Bq/\text{kg } fw)}{\text{Radionuclide activity concentration in feed } (Bq/\text{kg } dw)}$$

Transfer coefficient values can be derived by dividing a CR value by the daily dietary intake (in kg/d), and, conversely, CR values can be derived by multiplying the transfer coefficient value by the daily dietary intake (in kg/d). Over the last 40 years following the introduction of the transfer coefficient concept, many studies have been conducted to determine values for a range of radionuclide – animal product combinations.

To accurately estimate intake, both the dietary composition and relative contamination of each component (in *Bq*/kg dw) need to be quantified. Estimates of the feed intake of animals are more accurate in experimental studies under controlled conditions, whereas in field studies the intake is often not measured, which can lead to variability in reported F_f and F_m values.

The typical diet of agricultural animals varies between and within countries, and with the season according to feeding regimes (including whether the animals graze outdoors or are kept indoors), and is related to live weight, maintenance requirements and milk production rates. Regional data on animal nutrition requirements relevant to the region and farming system being considered can be used to derive dietary intake information. Preferably feed intake estimates would either be based on agricultural production criteria or acquired directly from the farming community. Grassy vegetation tends to be much more highly contaminated than other components of the diet, so all radionuclide intake can be assumed to come from this part of the diet when animals are consuming grass-based fodder. In published international cow milk datasets, some $\mathrm{F_m}$ and $\mathrm{F_f}$ values are based on estimated daily dry matter intake (DMI) many of which are best estimates or recommended values that do not take account of changes in the factors discussed above. Although the lack of measured daily DMI introduces uncertainty, it is unlikely to change derived $\mathrm{F_m}$ values by more than a factor of 3.

Transfer coefficients of radionuclides to milk and meat are generally lower for large animals, such as cattle, than for small animals, such as sheep, goats and hens. However, this is a side effect of the definition of the $\mathrm{F_m}$ and $\mathrm{F_f}$ because transfer coefficients incorporate daily DMI which increases with animal size. A higher $\mathrm{F_m}$ or $\mathrm{F_f}$ value does not mean that animal products from small animals will be more highly contaminated than those from larger animals, as was mistakenly reported in the past.

An alternative, simpler, approach to quantify transfer is to remove the dietary intake used in the estimation of $\mathrm{F_m}$ and calculate the CR – the equilibrium ratio between the radionuclide activity concentration in the animal food product (Bq/kg fw) divided by the radionuclide activity concentration in the feedstuff ingested (Bq/kg dw) (Howard et al. 2009a, b, 2016b; Smith and Beresford 2005). For most radionuclides, the compiled CR data gives similar values between different livestock species; therefore those derived for one species could be applied to another, providing a more generic parameter than the transfer coefficient. The advantage, especially for field studies, is that daily DMI does not need to be calculated or a value assumed. To apply CR values when a number of different feed types are consumed suggests that the relative proportions of each dietary component need to be known. However, if the grassy component is the main source of radionuclide contamination (which is normally the case), then the intake from other components, especially if imported, can be discounted.

Tables of available CR and Tag values for various animal products are provided for radionuclides in TRS 472 (IAEA 2010) and are discussed in more detail in TECDOC 1616 (IAEA 2009). More recent analysis of transfer parameters for goat and cow milk is provided in Howard et al. (2016b, 2017). Using available CR geometric mean values given in these two papers, the predicted radionuclide activity concentrations at equilibrium have been calculated for feed that contains 1000 Bg/kg dw. The figures show the considerable difference in transfer to milk and meat for different radionuclides. For cow milk (Fig. 5.2), the relatively high transfer of I, Cs and Sr is evident, and U is also high although there are only seven reported values for this radionuclide and therefore less confidence in the value. For meat the transfer of Cs and I is also relatively high. There is no data for Sr probably because transfer to these products is low and not a cause for concern (Fig. 5.3). Furthermore, other radionuclides may be important for meat, notably S, U and Co. Notably, Po, which is an alpha emitter, has mid-range CR values for both milk and meat although based on relatively few data.

The aggregated transfer coefficient is often used to quantify radionuclide transfer in non-intensive systems (termed a Tag, with units of m^2/kg) especially for animals and animal products. Tag is equal to the plant mass or animal tissue activity concentration (Bq/kg dw or fw) per unit area deposition density in the soil (Bq/m^2). Tag values are easier to apply in the emergency response and the transition phases after a NRE as authorities will probably initially report contamination in deposition density units of Bq/m^2. Tag were first proposed as more suitable for game animals after the Chernobyl NRE (Howard et al. 1991, 1996a, b). The determination of the

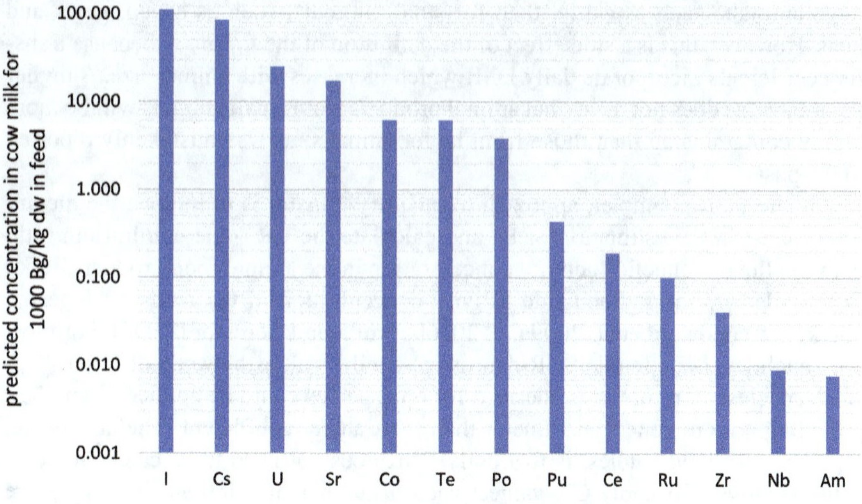

Fig. 5.2 Predicted activity concentrations of some radionuclides in cow milk from dairy cows given feed that contains 1000 Bg/kg dw. Note the plot uses a logarithmic axis

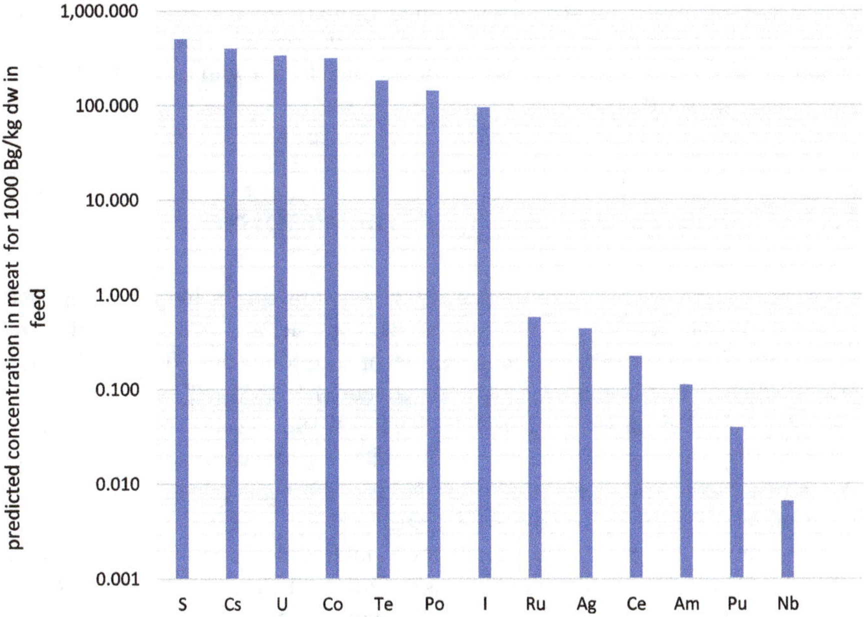

Fig. 5.3 Predicted activity concentrations of some radionuclides in meat for animals given feed that contains 1000 Bg/kg dw. Note the plot uses a logarithmic axis

underlying data for the deposition to soil needed to estimate aggregated transfer coefficients (Tag) (Howard et al. 1991, 1996a, b) is a key component in the use of the Tag value. The spatial resolution of the data is limited, and the animals considered have different sizes of home range from which they derive their food, which introduces an averaging effect but unavoidably includes uncertainties.

The use of Tag amalgamates a large number of underlying processes and is inevitably less precise than other measures described above that can be used if dietary intake is known or can be reliably estimated. Tag values rather than CR values are commonly used for free-ranging animals and for game animals in forested areas. Tag values are provided for some radionuclides in TRS 472 (IAEA 2010) and are discussed in more detail in TECDOC 1616 (IAEA 2009).

5.2.9 *Quantification of the Time Dependency of Radionuclide Activity Concentrations in Animal Products*

Assessments of the transfer of radionuclides via the human food chain are often based on equilibrium models using the parameter values given above. Such parameter values have limitations as they are not directly applicable to dynamic situations such as that which occurs after a NRE when radionuclide activity concentrations can change rapidly in the first few days or weeks. Once the release of radionuclides ceases, radionuclide activity concentrations in animals and animal products decline with time. Models that simulate the dynamic accumulation and excretion of radionuclides in farm animals and animal products often use biological half-lives $\left(T^{b}_{1/2}\right)$ combined with F_f, F_m or CR values to estimate the change with time (IAEA 2009; Brown and Simmonds 1995).

5.2.10 *Biological Half-Life ($T^{b}_{1/2}$) in Animal Tissues*

It is important to have some knowledge of the rate of loss from animals of ingested (or inhaled) radionuclides released after NREs. $T^{b}_{1/2}$values are used to quantify how quickly agricultural or other animals will become decontaminated if they are fed uncontaminated feed or removed from the contaminated area. $T^{b}_{1/2}$is defined as the time it takes for a given activity concentration in a tissue or an animal product, such as muscle, thyroid or milk, to reduce to half of its original activity concentration by processes excluding physical decay. $T^{b}_{1/2}$values have been compiled in tables for different animal products by Fesenko et al. (2015).

$T^{b}_{1/2}$ for milk are normally described using a single exponential function. For cow milk, $T^{b}_{1/2}$ values for different radionuclides are similar at about 2 days after a single administration (Fesenko et al. 2015). For all radionuclides considered, the $T^{b}_{1/2}$varied within a narrow range of 0.6–3.5 days with the shortest values for ^{131}I and ^{132}Te. The key message is that if grazing animals are removed from contaminated areas, or given uncontaminated (clean) feed, the radionuclide contamination of the milk will rapidly decline. If animals have been eating contaminated feed for a number of weeks, the rate of reduction in milk may be slower due to release and redistribution of radionuclides retained in different tissues.

There is variation in $T^{b}_{1/2}$ values due to age, species and tissues. Some differences occur because metabolic rate decreases with increasing body size. The $T^{b}_{1/2}$ tends to be longer for larger animals. For example, ^{137}Cs loss from muscle is faster for small ruminants such as sheep and goats than for larger ruminants such as cattle. Compiled $T^{b}_{1/2}$ values for muscle of cattle reported by Fesenko et al. (2015) for isotopes of Sr, Cs and I are summarized in Table 5.4. The loss is best described by two exponential components. Data for other tissues and agricultural animals are summarized in this publication.

Table 5.4 Range of values for biological half-lives of radionuclide activity concentrations and fraction of loss of radionuclide in the first component in muscles of cattle

		Biological half lives	
Radionuclide	Fraction of loss of radionuclide in the first component	Fast loss	Slow loss
^{90}Sr	0.42–0.9	3.0–4.0	180–700
^{131}I	1.0	7.0	
^{137}Cs	0.37–0.93	3.0–22.3	36.3–81

Summarized from Fesenko et al. (2015)

Losses of radionuclides from soft tissues tend to be shorter than those from bone (Fesenko et al. 2015). The $T_{1/2}^{b}$ values are relatively short for ^{132}Te, ^{137}Cs and ^{106}Ru, whereas they are longer if the radionuclides associate with proteins or colloids (e.g. ^{144}Ce). The longest $T_{1/2}^{b}$ values are for radionuclides which are deposited in bone, notably plutonium, americium and ^{90}Sr with half-life of 600–3100 days in cattle. Animals and animal products often have fast and slow components of retention in tissues that are described by double exponential functions.

Some tissues which accumulate certain elements (and their radioisotopes) for metabolic requirements need to retain the elements and, consequently, have long $T_{1/2}^{b}$ values. Key examples are thyroid which accumulates iodine (and, therefore, radioisotopes of iodine such as ^{131}I) and bone which accumulates Ca and its analogue ^{90}Sr.

5.2.11 Ecological and Effective Half-Lives

The long-term time-dependent behaviour of radionuclides in animal tissues can also be quantified using ecological or effective half-lives which integrates all biological, environmental and ecological processes that cause a decrease of radionuclide activity concentrations in an animal product.

The ecological half-life, $T_{1/2}^{eco}$, describes the reduction of amount of radionuclide (Bq) or activity concentration (Bq/kg) in a specific environmental medium. The ecological half-life for animal products is equal to the time required for the radionuclide activity concentration in a target specific animal tissue (or milk) to decrease by a factor of 2. It does not include the effects of physical radioactive decay of an isotope. Instead of estimating, $T_{1/2}^{eco}$, from radionuclide activity concentrations, the analysis can also be applied to transfer parameters described above such as the CR or the Tag.

Effective half-lives are derived when the reduction in activity concentration, CR or Tag due to physical decay has been considered in the data. The effective half-life ($T_{1/2}^{eff}$) is defined as the time required to lose half of the radionuclide activity concentration (or the value of a transfer parameter) in the target (such as an animal tissue) and is a result of the interrelation between the physical ($T_{1/2}^{p}$) and biological ($T_{1/2}^{b}$) half-lives. The $T_{1/2}^{eff}$ can be calculated according to the following equation:

$$T_{1/2}^{eff} = \left(T_{1/2}^{p} \times T_{1/2}^{b}\right) / \left(T_{1/2}^{p} + T_{1/2}^{b}\right)$$

For ^{131}I which has a $T_{1/2}^{p}$ of 8 days and, for example, a $T_{1/2}^{b}$ of 138 days, the $T_{1/2}^{eff}$ can be calculated as:

$$T_{1/2}^{eff} = (8 \times 138) / (8 + 138) = 1104 / 146 = 7.6\text{days}.$$

Long-term time series data of radiocaesium and radiostrontium activity concentrations in animal products can be used to provide such values. The data for changes with time are fitted with either a single or double exponential giving either a single

$T_{1/2}^{eff}$ or two $T_{1/2}^{eff}$ with an estimate of the proportion of loss that can be attributed to each component.

There are three prime sources of information on radionuclide half-lives in animal products: the Kyshtym and Chernobyl NREs and global fallout.

After the Chernobyl NPP NRE, there was a short-duration release with well-known characteristics, high contamination levels and varying environmental characteristics (such as soil and climate). As a result, extensive data on the changes with time of ^{137}Cs in animals have been obtained. Although the Fukushima NRE was also a relatively short-pulse release, there were few data for animals and animal products reported due to the disruption caused by the tsunami and earthquake and the relatively low importance of animal products because many agricultural animals were housed.

Global fallout represented a variable source term of radionuclides for the environment, as deposition of radionuclides occurred over a number of years, with maximum deposition observed in 1962–1964. A decade after the peak deposition period, when external contamination of plants was no longer occurring, long-term monitoring data provided an opportunity for deriving long-term effective half-lives for ^{90}Sr and ^{137}Cs.

5.3 Monitoring Animal Food Products

Monitoring the presence of radioactivity entering the food chain is of prime importance to ensure the safety of animal products reaching the human consumer. Milk is a major constituent of the diet for children, and the presence of ^{90}Sr, ^{131}I and ^{137}Cs needs to be carefully assessed. Regular examination of dairy and agricultural produce has been an important role of the veterinary and relevant authorities in many countries for many years. For example, milk in Europe is routinely analysed from the vicinity of nuclear sites to assess the exposure from ingested foodstuffs to the local population. The NREs at Chernobyl and Fukushima Daiichi intensified surveillance globally.

After NREs, national monitoring programmes have been implemented and maps of the deposition of radioactive contamination prepared. The strategies for monitoring need to adapt to the changing characteristics of contamination that occur with time. Initially, ^{131}I is potentially the major hazard in milk, after which monitoring for ^{137}Cs in milk and meat is more likely to dominate. Therefore, sampling of milk from contaminated areas is given a high priority. Fortunately, collection and analysis of milk is much easier for ^{131}I and radiocaesium than for other animal products. Analysis of milk from individual farms will give detailed information about the extent and character of the contamination. However, there is also some advantage in sampling milk from bulk sources such as tankers, which gives data representing several hundred cows sourced from a wide area.

If the radionuclide activity concentration in an animal product is above the intervention level, management options such as decontamination by clean feeding, or administration of Cs binders, which reduce its absorption in the gut, can be used to lower the activity concentration before slaughter (see management options and datasheets). The time period needed to do this can be assessed based on measured radionuclide activity concentrations in muscle and the corresponding radiation safety standard (intervention level), utilizing knowledge of $T^b_{1/2}$.

The use of live monitoring reduces the need to condemn meat and provides important information on the effectiveness of options which aim to reduce contamination of animals. Live monitoring has been used extensively after the Chernobyl NRE in both the USSR (subsequently termed the former Soviet Union (fSU) countries) and Western Europe to measure radiocaesium in a wide range of live ruminants and also for carcasses of wild animals to inform hunters of the contamination levels in the meat. The advantage of live monitoring is that estimates of radiocaesium activity concentrations can be made without the need to slaughter the animal. Live monitoring was less widely used after the Fukushima NRE due to the relatively low radiocaesium activity concentrations. Blood sampling and analysis was also used to assess animal product contamination.

5.4 Radionuclide Transfer to Intensively Farmed Agricultural Animals

Although many different radionuclides may be released in a NRE, only a few present potentially serious health hazards to humans and animals. There are three key radionuclides: radioiodine, radiocaesium and radiostrontium, which are environmentally mobile in many production systems and which transfer readily to animal products. Because of their importance, specific text on these three radionuclides is included for each subsection describing environmental transfer rates below.

This section describes various factors which influence radionuclide transfer in intensively managed systems which are normally fertilized, and where the farm animals are in a good condition with high milk and meat production rates. Data for CR are provided in tables for different radionuclides and animal products based on compilations that were published by the IAEA (which used the term Transfer factor) in IAEA (2009, 2010).

5.4.1 Soil and Plant Aspects

Soil is the main terrestrial sink of long-lived radionuclides deposited on the landscape, so the interaction between radionuclides and different soil characteristics is particularly important after the initial phase. In some cases, a substantial proportion of the radionuclide may become strongly associated with soil components and thereby becomes less mobile.

5.4.1.1 Radioiodine

The geochemistry of iodine is dominated by its volatility. The volatilization of organo-iodine compounds and elemental iodine from biological and non-biological sources in the oceans is a major component of its global cycle. Iodine is strongly enriched in soils 50–80 km inland from marine systems. Some wetland soils also form terrestrial sources of volatilized iodine. The dominant species of iodine in the aerobic soil environment are I^-, IO_3^- and I_2.

Stable ^{127}I is normally present in soils at an average concentration of 5 mg/kg dw. Typically, terrestrial plants and food crops contain from 0.07 to 10 mg/kg dw of stable I (^{127}I). There is another natural isotope of iodine, ^{129}I, that is much less abundant and which can be released during some nuclear activities, including NREs, but has a much lower radiological impact than ^{131}I.

Radioiodine dissolves in water and moves easily from the atmosphere into different components of the environment. However, it readily absorbs to various soil components such as organic matter and soil minerals which limits the uptake of iodine through the plant root system. The two naturally occurring isotopes usually behave similarly although soil to plant uptake rates have been shown to differ in some soils (IAEA 2009).

The importance of soil to plant transfer for short-lived radioiodine isotopes, especially ^{131}I, is generally thought to be negligible because of the short physical half-life of the iodine isotopes of relevance for internal dose to humans. After NRE, the interception by plants of the short-lived ^{131}I in the emergency and transition phase is important, but in the longer term, accumulation of iodine in plants is only relevant for ^{129}I.

The transfer of radioiodine from soil to plant in the emergency phase after NREs has received little attention from the research and radiation protection community. There are few compiled data for iodine transfer to plants (Table 5.5) with CR values varying from 0.1 to 5.0 for vegetative plant mass. No CR values for iodine are given for soil to grass species in TRS 472 (IAEA 2010). CR values for iodine are low for soils with a high cation exchange capacity and organic matter content. For grain (rye and wheat), which can be components of animals' diet, iodine CR values vary from 5×10^{-4} to 8×10^{-3}.

Table 5.5 Soil to plant transfer factors for I (IAEA 2009, 2010)[a]

Plant group	Plant compartment	Soil group	N	GM	Minimum	Maximum
Cereal	Grain	All	13	6.3×10^{-4}	1.0×10^{-4}	1.1×10^{-2}
		Clay	6	5.7×10^{-4}	2.0×10^{-4}	1.6×10^{-3}
		Loam	5	3.6×10^{-4}	1.0×10^{-4}	1.2×10^{-3}
		Sand	2		1.0×10^{-3}	1.1×10^{-2}
Leafy vegetables	Leaves	All	12	6.5×10^{-3}	1.1×10^{-3}	1.0×10^{-1}
		Clay	2	4.6×10^{-3}	1.6×10^{-3}	1.3×10^{-2}
		Loam	8	4.1×10^{-3}	1.1×10^{-3}	8.0×10^{-3}
		Sand	1			

(continued)

Table 5.5 (continued)

Plant group	Plant compartment	Soil group	N	GM	Minimum	Maximum
Nonleafy vegetables	Head, berries, buds	All	1	1.0×10^{-1}		
Leguminous vegetables	Seeds and pod	All	23	8.5×10^{-3}	2.0×10^{-4}	1.4×10^{-1}
		Clay	2		2.0×10^{-4}	3.0×10^{-4}
		Loam	3	4.4×10^{-4}	3.0×10^{-4}	7.0×10^{-4}
		Sand	2		3.3×10^{-3}	3.7×10^{-3}
Root crops	Root	All	28	7.7×10^{-3}	1.4×10^{-3}	4.7×10^{-2}
		Clay	7	4.5×10^{-3}	1.4×10^{-3}	2.8×10^{-2}
		Loam	12	4.7×10^{-3}	1.5×10^{-3}	1.6×10^{-2}
		Sand	9	2.3×10^{-2}	1.2×10^{-2}	4.7×10^{-2}
Tubers	Tuber	All	1			
Pasture	Stems, leaves	All	12	3.7×10^{-3}	9.0×10^{-4}	5.0×10^{-1}
		Clay	2		8.4×10^{-3}	9.0×10^{-3}
		Sand	9	1.8×10^{-3}	9.0×10^{-4}	8.5×10^{-3}
Cereal	Stems, leaves	All	16	5.2×10^{-2}	7.0×10^{-3}	7.5×10^{-1}
		Clay	7	4.5×10^{-2}	1.0×10^{-2}	1.9×10^{-1}
		Loam	7	3.6×10^{-2}	7.0×10^{-3}	2.0×10^{-1}
		Sand	2		1.1×10^{-1}	7.5×10^{-1}

[a] N - sample number, GM - goemetric mean - The mean is a geometric mean except where the number of data values (N) is less than 3, in which case it is an arithmetic mean. Further statistical information is given for a wider range of radionuclides in TECDOC 1616 and TRS 472 (IAEA 2009, 2010)

5.4.1.2 Radiocaesium

Radiocaesium has a high biological and ecological mobility as stable caesium is an alkali element, which is a chemical analogue of the biologically important element, potassium. Stable caesium exists in the environment in the 1+ oxidation state with concentrations ranging between 0.3 and 25 mg/kg dw. Radiocaesium is highly mobile in soils of both agricultural and free-ranging farming and harvesting systems in the emergency phase after NRE deposition.

In the transition phase and the subsequent existing exposure situation, after radiocaesium has been lost from the surfaces of plants, root uptake of radiocaesium from soil dominates. During the year following the Chernobyl NRE, the ^{137}Cs activity concentration in plants declined by a factor of between 3 and 100 as root uptake from different soil types became the dominant contamination route. The most important process controlling plant root uptake of radiocaesium is the interaction between soil matrix and soil solution which depends primarily on the cation exchange capacity of the soil. For mineral soils, this is influenced by the concentrations and types of clay minerals and the concentrations of competitive major cations, especially potassium and ammonium. The extent of selective, irreversible absorption differs for different clay minerals. Sorption of caesium to organic colloids and dissolved organic matter is not important in most (but not all) soils, so caesium is relatively more mobile in peaty and sandy soils. Organic soils often contain sufficient illitic clay minerals to immobilize radiocaesium present in organic soils, but the organic matter holds the clay in an expanded state, thereby maintaining availability of radiocaesium for plant uptake (Hird et al. 1995).

Accumulation of radiocaesium into crops and pasture is related to soil texture. On sandy soils, uptake of radiocaesium by plants is approximately twice as high as on loam soils mainly due to the lower concentrations of potassium in sand. Radiocaesium uptake from poor, often unfertilized, soils tends to exceed that of plants grown on fertile agricultural soils by several orders of magnitude. The highest ^{137}Cs uptake by roots from soil to plants occurs in poor highly organic, boggy soils, which are one to two orders of magnitude higher than in sandy soils. Agricultural practices often reduce the transfer of radionuclides from soils to plant by physical dilution (e.g. ploughing) or by adding competitive elements during normal fertilization procedures. For radiocaesium, application of its analogue, potassium, is highly effective in reducing transfer to crops.

In TRS 472 (IAEA 2010), CR values for caesium have been given for a wide range of different plant groups (Table 5.6). Caesium uptake from soil by a single crop is less than 0.1% of the soil's content (Menzel 1963). CR values vary considerably from about 10^{-3} up to about 1.0. Variations in the accumulation of ^{137}Cs by plants due to differences in soil properties are up to a factor of 100, and the effect of biological features of plants causes up to a further tenfold variation (Alexakhin and Korneyev 1991). Mean caesium CR values are a factor of 2–10 lower than those of

Table 5.6 Soil to plant for Cs (IAEA 2009, 2010)[a]

Plant group	Plant compartment	Soil group	N	GM	Minimum	Maximum
Cereal	Grain	All	470	2.9×10^{-2}	2.0×10^{-4}	9.0×10^{-1}
		Clay	110	1.1×10^{-2}	2.0×10^{-4}	9.0×10^{-2}
		Loam	158	2.0×10^{-2}	8.0×10^{-4}	2.0×10^{-1}
		Sand	156	3.9×10^{-2}	2.0×10^{-3}	6.6×10^{-1}
		Organic	28	4.3×10^{-2}	1.0×10^{-2}	7.3×10^{-1}
Maize	Grain	All	67	3.3×10^{-2}	3.0×10^{-3}	2.6×10^{-1}
		Clay	11	1.2×10^{-2}	3.0×10^{-3}	7.0×10^{-2}
		Loam	14	1.6×10^{-2}	3.2×10^{-3}	7.0×10^{-2}
		Sand	47	4.9×10^{-2}	8.0×10^{-3}	2.6×10^{-1}
Leafy vegetables	Leaves	All	290	6.0×10^{-2}	3.0×10^{-4}	9.8×10^{-1}
		Clay	67	1.8×10^{-2}	5.0×10^{-4}	7.2×10^{-1}
		Loam	119	7.4×10^{-2}	3.0×10^{-4}	7.3×10^{-1}
		Sand	96	1.2×10^{-1}	2.1×10^{-3}	9.8×10^{-1}
		Organic	7	2.25×10^{-2}	4.0×10^{-3}	4.6×10^{-1}
Nonleafy vegetables	Head, berries, buds	All	38	2.1×10^{-2}	7.0×10^{-4}	7.3×10^{-1}
		Clay	14	9.1×10^{-3}	7.0×10^{-4}	1.6×10^{-2}
		Loam	5	3.3×10^{-2}	6.3×10^{-3}	3.0×10^{-1}
		Sand	17	3.5×10^{-2}	1.2×10^{-2}	7.3×10^{-1}
Leguminous vegetables	Seeds and pod	All	126	4.0×10^{-2}	1.0×10^{-3}	7.1×10^{-1}
		Clay	18	1.3×10^{-2}	2.0×10^{-3}	8.1×10^{-2}
		Loam	42	2.0×10^{-2}	1.0×10^{-3}	4.2×10^{-1}
		Sand	66	8.7×10^{-2}	3.5×10^{-3}	7.1×10^{-1}

(continued)

Table 5.6 (continued)

Plant group	Plant compartment	Soil group	N	GM	Minimum	Maximum
Root crops	Root	All	81	4.2×10^{-2}	1.0×10^{-3}	8.8×10^{-1}
		Clay	17	2.4×10^{-2}	5.0×10^{-3}	6.0×10^{-2}
		Loam	21	3.0×10^{-2}	1.0×10^{-3}	1.6×10^{-1}
		Sand	37	6.2×10^{-2}	8.0×10^{-3}	4.0×10^{-1}
		Organic	5	5.9×10^{-2}	1.6×10^{-2}	8.8×10^{-1}
Tubers	Tuber	All	138	5.6×10^{-2}	4.0×10^{-3}	6.0×10^{-1}
		Clay	21	2.5×10^{-2}	5.0×10^{-3}	9.0×10^{-2}
		Loam	40	3.5×10^{-2}	4.8×10^{-3}	1.4×10^{-1}
		Sand	69	9.3×10^{-2}	4.0×10^{-3}	6.0×10^{-1}
		Organic	7	5.8×10^{-2}	1.610^{-2}	5.4×10^{-1}
Grasses	Stems, leaves	All	64	6.3×10^{-2}	4.8×10^{-3}	9.9×10^{-1}
		Clay	9	1.2×10^{-2}	4.8×10^{-3}	4.3×10^{-2}
		Loam	10	4.8×10^{-2}	1.2×10^{-2}	2.1×10^{-1}
		Sand	41	8.4×10^{-2}	1.0×10^{-2}	9.9×10^{-1}
		Organic	4	2.8×10^{-1}	2.1×10^{-1}	3.4×10^{-1}
Fodder leguminous	Stems, leaves	All	85	1.6×10^{-1}	1.0×10^{-2}	1.8
		Clay	4	4.6×10^{-2}	1.3×10^{-2}	3.0×10^{-1}
		Loam	51	1.5×10^{-1}	1.0×10^{-2}	1.2
		Sand	29	2.4×10^{-1}	1.8×10^{-2}	1.8
Pasture	Stems, leaves	All	401	2.5×10^{-1}	1.0×10^{-2}	5.0
		Clay	75	1.8×10^{-1}	1.0×10^{-2}	1.2
		Loam	124	1.9×10^{-1}	1.0×10^{-2}	2.6
		Sand	169	2.9×10^{-1}	1.0×10^{-2}	4.8
		Organic	31	7.6×10^{-1}	3.0×10^{-1}	5.0
Herbs	Stems, leaves	All	4	6.6×10^{-2}	4.8×10^{-3}	2.8
Other crops		All	9	3.1×10^{-1}	3.6×10^{-2}	2.2
Cereal	Stems, leaves	All	130	1.5×10^{-1}	4.3×10^{-3}	3.7
		Clay	37	5.6×10^{-2}	4.3×10^{-3}	5.3×10^{-1}
		Loam	36	1.1×10^{-1}	6.5×10^{-3}	1.5
		Sand	35	2.1×10^{-1}	4.1×10^{-2}	1.9
Maize	Stems, leaves	All	101	7.3×10^{-2}	3.0×10^{-3}	4.9×10^{-1}
		Clay	11	2.2×10^{-2}	7.8×10^{-3}	6.0×10^{-2}
		Loam	10	1.5×10^{-2}	3.0×10^{-3}	5.2×10^{-2}
		Sand	77	1.0×10^{-1}	1.4×10^{-2}	4.9×10^{-1}
		Organic	3	1.4×10^{-1}	1.0×10^{-1}	1.6×10^{-1}
Root crops	Leaves	All	12	3.5×10^{-2}	6.0×10^{-3}	4.5×10^{-1}
		Clay	7	2.6×10^{-2}	6.0×10^{-3}	4.7×10^{-2}
		Loam	2		9.0×10^{-3}	4.3×10^{-2}
		Sand	3	1.1×10^{-1}	5.1×10^{-2}	4.5×10^{-1}

[a] The mean is a geometric mean except where the number of data values (N) is less than 3, in which case it is an arithmetic mean. Further statistical information is given for a wider range of radionuclides in TECDOC 1616 and TRS 472 (IAEA 2009, 2010)

Table 5.7 Radioecological sensitivity for soil-plant transfer of $^{137}Cs/^{134}Cs$

Sensitivity	Soil characteristic	Mechanism	Example
High	– Low nutrient content – Very low fraction of clay minerals – High organic content	– Little competition with potassium and ammonium in root uptake	Peat soils
Medium	– Poor nutrient status, consisting of minerals including some clays	– Limited competition with potassium and ammonium during root uptake	Podzol, other sandy soils
Low	– High nutrient status – High fraction of clay minerals	– Radiocaesium strongly bound to clay minerals – Strong competition with potassium and ammonium during root uptake	Chernozems Clay and loam soils (used for intensive agriculture)

strontium in most soils. The radioecological sensitivity of soils for radiocaesium can be broadly divided into the categories listed in Table 5.7.

A substantial proportion of the radiocaesium in soil gradually becomes less available for plant uptake as it becomes irreversibly bound by clay minerals. Differences in radioecological sensitivities of soils after the first few years can have a significant impact on animal production contamination after an NRE. In some areas with low radiocaesium deposition densities and highly radioecologically sensitive soils after the Chernobyl accident, there were high radiocaesium activity concentrations in plants, and hence animals, which persisted for decades. Conversely, some areas of high deposition with soils of low radioecological sensitivity for radiocaesium had only low to moderate radiocaesium activity concentrations in plants and animals.

5.4.1.3 Radiostrontium

Natural strontium consists of 4 stable isotopes with mass numbers of 84, 86, 87 and 88. The content of stable Sr in the Earth's crust is about $3 \times 10^{-2}\%$. The chemical properties of strontium are determined by its position in group 2 of the periodic system and are typical for alkali-earth elements. Strontium is a close analogue of calcium and its behaviour in soils and transfer to plants are highly influenced by the status of calcium in soils. Strontium is a highly mobile and bioavailable element that exists in the environment in the Sr(II) oxidation state at concentrations in soils that range between 50 and 1000 mg/kg dw. Strontium is usually present in the surface environment as a carbonate or a sulphate mineral. The dominant aqueous strontium species in natural waters over a broad pH range (2–9) is the free divalent Sr^{2+}. Cation exchange is the key mechanism of absorption of Sr in soil.

Strontium is one of the most biologically mobile elements. Plant crops take up about 0.2% to 3% of the strontium in the soil (Menzel 1963). The Kyshtym NRE was the first instance where large areas were contaminated by radionuclides, and ^{90}Sr was one of the most important radionuclides released. Therefore, there is a large amount of available information on the behaviour of radiostrontium in soils. The uptake of ^{90}Sr from soil to plants is affected by presence of both stable strontium and stable calcium (Gulyakin and Yudintseva 1962, Arkhipov et al. 1969). The interaction with these two stable elements is one of the main contributors to variability in Sr CR values. Strontium uptake by plants is generally highest from soils of low calcium content and, in many cases, of high organic matter content.

A large number of CR values are reported for Sr in TRS 472 (IAEA 2010) which are summarized in Table 5.8. Strontium CR values differ by more than a factor of 100, depending on soil properties and biological features of plants. Most of the variation in CR values of ^{90}Sr can be attributed to the stable strontium concentrations in soil and its interaction with calcium. These two factors largely account for the low CR values, and also the large variability reported between individual plant

Table 5.8 Soil to plant transfer factors for Sr[a]

Plant group	Plant compartment	Soil group	N	GM	Minimum	Maximum
Cereal	Grain	All	282	1.1×10^{-1}	3.6×10^{-3}	1.0
		Clay	72	7.8×10^{-2}	5.3×10^{-3}	7.1×10^{-1}
		Loam	71	1.1×10^{-1}	1.6×10^{-2}	7.2×10^{-1}
		Sand	123	1.4×10^{-1}	3.6×10^{-3}	1.0
		Organic	10	9.7×10^{-2}	1.2×10^{-2}	3.6×10^{-1}
Maize	Grain	All	39	3.2×10^{-1}	2.0×10^{-3}	2.6
		Clay	7	6.9×10^{-2}	2.0×10^{-3}	3.9×10^{-1}
		Loam	13	3.6×10^{-1}	1.5×10^{-1}	8.6×10^{-1}
		Sand	19	5.2×10^{-1}	4.0×10^{-2}	2.6
Leafy vegetables	Leaves	All	217	7.6×10^{-1}	3.9×10^{-3}	7.8
		Clay	54	1.5×10^{-1}	3.9×10^{-3}	2.2
		Loam	84	1.2	4.1×10^{-2}	5.0
		Sand	72	1.7	6.4×10^{-2}	7.8
		Organic	6	2.1×10^{-1}	1.5×10^{-1}	3.0×10^{-1}
Nonleafy vegetables	Head, berries, buds	All	19	3.6×10^{-1}	7.1×10^{-3}	7.9
		Clay	8	1.3×10^{-1}	7.1×10^{-3}	8.6×10^{-1}
		Loam	3	1.4	9.0×10^{-1}	2.3
		Sand	5	8.7×10^{-1}	2.0×10^{-1}	7.9
		Organic	2	2.2×10^{-1}	1.9×10^{-1}	2.5×10^{-1}
Leguminous vegetables	Seeds and pod	All	148	1.4	1.3×10^{-1}	6.0
		Clay	25	6.2×10^{-1}	1.3×10^{-1}	2.6
		Loam	68	1.3	1.7×10^{-1}	4.6
		Sand	55	2.2	3.0×10^{-1}	6.0
Root crops	Root	All	56	7.2×10^{-1}	3.0×10^{-2}	4.8
		Clay	13	4.1×10^{-1}	5.2×10^{-2}	3.9
		Loam	16	6.1×10^{-1}	4.4×10^{-2}	4.5
		Sand	26	1.1	3.0×10^{-2}	4.8

(continued)

Table 5.8 (continued)

Plant group	Plant compartment	Soil group	N	GM	Minimum	Maximum
Tubers	Tuber	All	106	1.6×10^{-1}	7.4×10^{-3}	1.6
		Clay	21	1.3×10^{-1}	2.6×10^{-2}	6.7×10^{-1}
		Loam	41	1.3×10^{-1}	7.4×10^{-3}	4.5×10^{-1}
		Sand	39	2.2×10^{-1}	2.6×10^{-2}	1.6
		Organic	4	5.8×10^{-2}	8.0×10^{-3}	2.3×10^{-1}
Grasses	Stems, leaves	All	50	9.1×10^{-1}	2.5×10^{-1}	2.8
		Clay	7	7.9×10^{-1}	4.8×10^{-1}	9.7×10^{-1}
		Loam	6	6.0×10^{-1}	2.9×10^{-1}	2.0
		Sand	34	1.1	2.6×10^{-1}	2.8
		Organic	3	2.6×10^{-1}	2.5×10^{-1}	2.8×10^{-1}
Fodder leguminous	Stems, leaves	All	35	3.7	1.3	1.8×10
		Clay	10	2.8	1.3	5.8
		Loam	11	3.3	1.4	9.8
		Sand	14	4.9	1.3	1.8×10
		Organic	1	3.9×10^{-1}		
Pasture	Stems, leaves	All	172	1.3	5.6×10^{-2}	7.3
		Clay	22	8.0×10^{-1}	9.0×10^{-2}	2.8
		Loam	58	1.1	3.7×10^{-1}	2.6
		Sand	87	1.7	9.8×10^{-2}	7.3
		Organic	4	3.5×10^{-1}	5.6×10^{-2}	1.2
Herbs	Stems, leaves	All	1	4.5		
Other crops		All	9	8.8×10^{-1}	2.0×10^{-2}	8.2
Cereal	Stems, leaves	All	37	1.1	1.5×10^{-1}	9.8
		Clay	20	7.5×10^{-1}	1.5×10^{-1}	2.8
		Loam	3	1.8	7.2×10^{-1}	3.6
		Sand	11	2.1	9.3×10^{-1}	9.8
Maize	Stems, leaves	All	36	7.3×10^{-1}	1.2×10^{-1}	3.0
		Clay	6	5.0×10^{-1}	1.8×10^{-1}	1.1
		Loam	7	7.0×10^{-1}	2.8×10^{-1}	1.4
		Sand	23	8.2×10^{-1}	1.2×10^{-1}	3.0

[a] The mean is a geometric mean except where the number of data values (N) is less than 3, in which case it is an arithmetic mean. Further statistical information is given for a wider range of radionuclides in TECDOC 1616 and TRS 472 (IAEA 2009, 2010)

types, which are affected by the need and ability to accumulate calcium. The radioecological sensitivity of soils for radiostrontium can be broadly divided into two categories listed in Table 5.9.

Decrease in exchangeable strontium in soil occurs very slowly, so the availability of soil ^{90}Sr to plants decreases only slightly with time. Relatively higher rates of ^{90}Sr vertical migration occur in sandy soils and lower rates in peat soils.

Table 5.9 Radioecological sensitivity for soil-plant transfer of ^{90}Sr

Sensitivity	Soil characteristic	Mechanism	Example
High	Low nutrient status Low organic matter content	Limited competition with calcium in root uptake	Podzol sandy soils
Low	High nutrient status Medium to high organic matter content	Strong competition with calcium in root uptake	Umbric gley soils, peaty soils

5.4.1.4 Other Radionuclides

Brief information is provided here on the other radionuclides of potential concern after an NRE based on text from IAEA TRS 472 (IAEA 2010) and TECDOC 1616 (IAEA 2009). Further, more detailed information, including CR values, can be accessed in these publications.

Transuranic elements (Am, Cm, Pu, Np) exhibit a complex soil chemistry, because of various degrees of oxidation, absence of stable carriers and high tendencies to complexation and hydrolysis. CR values for transuranic elements vary from about 100 to about 10^{-6}. Due to these relatively low CR values, the activity concentrations of these radionuclides in fruits and grains are 10–1000 times lower than in the vegetative parts of plants. Accumulation of these elements decreases in the order Np > Am > Cm > Pu. Hydrolysis is a major factor influencing the behaviour of Am and Cm in soils. The mobility of Pu depends on its valency form and decreases in the order Pu (V) > Pu (VI) > Pu (III) > Pu (IV).

The fission products (^{89}Sr, ^{90}Sr, ^{134}Cs, ^{137}Cs, ^{129}I, ^{131}I, ^{95}Zr, ^{95}Nb, ^{103}Ru, ^{106}Ru, ^{141}Ce, ^{144}Ce) include a diverse class of elements. Of these radionuclides, ^{95}Zr, ^{95}Nb, ^{103}Ru, ^{106}Ru and ^{141}Ce, ^{144}Ce are poorly accumulated by agricultural plants because of their strong sorption in soil, leading to low CR values. Soil pH and organic matter content are the most significant soil characteristics that influence the behaviour of these radionuclides. Up to 99% of the plant uptake of these radionuclides is retained in the roots, so there is little transfer to above-ground plant parts that may be consumed by animals. CR values vary by factors of 10–30 for different soils, with the lowest plant uptake for ^{95}Zr and ^{141}Ce, ^{144}Ce.

The activation products (^{60}Co, ^{65}Zn) are radioisotopes of biologically important microelements. They have high mobility in soil-plant systems and, therefore, relatively high CR values. In particular, ^{65}Zn has CR values from 1.0 to 15.0, but it is not likely to be released in large quantities after a NRE.

The behaviour of other radionuclides not mentioned above depends on the oxidation-reduction potential of the soil, the acidity of soil solution and the organic matter content.

5.4.2 *Dairy Production*

The consumption of milk contaminated by ^{131}I, ^{90}Sr and ^{137}Cs is potentially one of the main contributors to the internal dose to humans after a NRE.

The highest contamination levels in plants are normally reached during the urgent response phase when radionuclides are intercepted by plants and before they are lost from the plant surfaces. At the time of the Chernobyl NPP NRE, vegetation was at different growth stages in different countries that were affected depending on latitude and elevation. In the first few weeks, interception on plant leaves of dry deposition and atmospheric washout with precipitation were the main pathways of contamination. Because radionuclides were released over a period of 10 days, and plant growth had commenced in the adjacent areas (as it was late April and early May), radionuclides were intercepted by plant surfaces including pasture grass. In contrast, because the Fukushima Daiichi NRE occurred in mid-March, there was much less plant biomass present that could intercept the radionuclides in the atmosphere. Therefore, in the prevailing intensive farming systems, the initial extent of contamination of most plants was much lower than that after the Chernobyl NRE.

In the USSR, the food-production systems at the time of the Chernobyl NRE were largely collective farms and small private subsistence farms. The collective farms had an intensive farming approach using land rotation combined with ploughing and fertilization to improve productivity. In contrast, the traditional small subsistence or "private" farms usually had privately owned livestock which often grazed in forest clearings to which they applied manure to improve yield instead of artificial fertilizers. Root uptake of radiocaesium becomes the key transfer route to milk after the emergency response phase and the early part of the transition phase. The highest activity concentrations of radionuclides in most agricultural animal product foodstuffs occurred in the growing season of 1986. In many regions of the USSR, as well as in Germany, France and Southern Europe, dairy animals were already grazing outdoors, so some contamination of cow, goat and sheep milk occurred. In contrast, in Northern Europe, in the early spring, most dairy cows, sheep and goats were not yet on pasture; therefore, there was little milk contamination.

The extent of transfer of radionuclides into cow, sheep and goat milk has been reported as both F_m and CR values in the IAEA publications TECDOC 1616 and TRS 472 (IAEA 2009, 2010). The data for cow and goat milk has recently been updated during the IAEA MODARIA programme (Howard et al. 2016a, b, 2017). F_m and CR values for selected radionuclide elements that are most relevant for NRE in the MODARIA tables are shown in Tables 5.10 and 5.11 for cow milk and Tables 5.12 and 5.13 for goat milk, respectively. Available parameter values for other radionuclides/elements can be found in Howard et al. (Howard et al. 2016a, b, 2017).

For some radionuclides released from previous NREs, there are few data, notably for ^{210}Po and ^{95}Zr. Also, data for transuranic elements such as plutonium, americium

Table 5.10 Transfer coefficients (F_m, d/kg) for radionuclides relevant for NREs for cow milk

Element	N	GM	Minimum	Maximum
Am	3	1.6×10^{-6}	3.0×10^{-7}	3.0×10^{-5}
Ce	8	1.5×10^{-5}	1.0×10^{-6}	1.3×10^{-4}
Co	16	3.2×10^{-4}	2.2×10^{-5}	1.0×10^{-2}
Cs	289	4.9×10^{-3}	6.0×10^{-4}	5.7×10^{-2}
I	105	6.0×10^{-3}	4.0×10^{-4}	4.4×10^{-2}
Nb	1	4.1×10^{-7}		
Po	4	2.4×10^{-4}	1.2×10^{-4}	3.0×10^{-4}
Pu	3	3.6×10^{-5}	7.5×10^{-6}	5.0×10^{-4}
Ru	6	9.4×10^{-6}	6.7×10^{-7}	1.4×10^{-4}
Sr	118	1.3×10^{-3}	1.5×10^{-5}	4.3×10^{-3}
Te	11	3.2×10^{-4}	7.8×10^{-5}	1.0×10^{-3}
U	7	2.5×10^{-3}	5.0×10^{-4}	6.1×10^{-3}
Zr	6	3.6×10^{-6}	5.5×10^{-5}	1.7×10^{-5}

Howard et al. (2017)

Table 5.11 Concentration ratios (CR, kg/L) for radionuclides relevant for NREs for cow milk

Element	N	GM	Minimum	Maximum
Am	3	7.7×10^{-6}	6.2×10^{-6}	6.2×10^{-4}
Ce	8	1.9×10^{-4}	1.0×10^{-5}	3.2×10^{-3}
Co	16	6.1×10^{-3}	4.5×10^{-4}	2.4×10^{-1}
Cs	289	8.4×10^{-2}	3.6×10^{-3}	9×10^{-1}
I	105	1.1×10^{-1}	3.0×10^{-3}	1.1×10^{-1}
Nb	1	9.0×10^{-6}		
Po	4	3.8×10^{-3}	2.4×10^{-3}	5.4×10^{-3}
Pu	3	4.3×10^{-4}	5.8×10^{-5}	5.0×10^{-3}
Ru	6	1.0×10^{-4}	1.0×10^{-5}	1.4×10^{-3}
Sr	118	1.7×10^{-2}	5.6×10^{-4}	1.4×10^{-1}
Te	11	6.1×10^{-3}	1.4×10^{-3}	1.1×10^{-2}
U	7	2.5×10^{-2}	5.0×10^{-3}	6.1×10^{-2}
Zr	6	4.1×10^{-5}	1.0×10^{-5}	$1.7x10^{-4}$

Howard et al. (2017)

and uranium are sparse. However, there are a large number of data for the most important radionuclides, ^{134}Cs, ^{137}Cs, ^{90}Sr and ^{131}I, and, therefore, there is more confidence in these transfer parameter values. Various factors that lead to the variability in the transfer values, such as the effect of the intake of a close stable element analogue to a radionuclide, is discussed for the three most important radionuclide elements below.

Table 5.12 Transfer coefficients (F_m, d/kg) for radionuclides relevant for NREs for goat milk*

Element	N	AM	ASD	GM	GSD	Minimum	Maximum
Am	2	2.8×10^{-5}				3.7×10^{-6}	5.2×10^{-5}
Ce	1	4.0×10^{-5}					
Cs	27	1.4×10^{-1}	7.9×10^{-2}	1.1×10^{-1}	2.1	9.0×10^{-3}	3.3×10^{-1}
I	23	3.2×10^{-1}	2.3×10^{-1}	2.1×10^{-1}	3.0	2.7×10^{-2}	7.7×10^{-1}
Po	2	2.3×10^{-3}				1.8×10^{-3}	2.7×10^{-3}
S	12	4.7×10^{-2}	1.9×10^{-2}	3.8×10^{-2}	1.7	1.6×10^{-2}	6.8×10^{-2}
Sr	21	2.0×10^{-2}	1.9×10^{-2}	1.5×10^{-2}	2.0	5.8×10^{-3}	8.1×10^{-2}
Te	1	4.4×10^{-3}					
U	1	1.4×10^{-3}					
Zr	1	5.5×10^{-6}					

N Sample size, *AM* arithmetic mean, *ASD* arithmetic standard deviation, *GM* geometric mean, *GSD* geometric standard deviation,
Howard et al. (2016a, b)
*The mean is a geometric mean except where the number of data values (N) is less than 3, in which case it is a n arithmetic mean. Further statistical information is given for a wider range of radionuclides in TECDOC 1616 and TRS 472 (IAEA 2009, 2010)

Table 5.13 Concentration ratios (CR, kg/L) for radionuclides relevant for NREs for goat milk*

Element	N	AM	ASD	GM	GSD	Minimum	Maximum
Am	2	4.4×10^{-5}				4.4×10^{-6}	8.4×10^{-5}
Ce	1	6.4×10^{-5}					
Cs	26	2.2×10^{-2}	9.8×10^{-2}	2.0×10^{-1}	1.7	4.9×10^{-2}	4.3×10^{-1}
I	21	5.3×10^{-1}	4.0×10^{-1}	3.2×10^{-1}	3.1	4.4×10^{-2}	1.2×100
Po	2	3.6×10^{-3}				2.9×10^{-3}	4.3×10^{-3}
S	12	8.3×10^{-2}	3.9×10^{-2}	7.3×10^{-2}	1.7	3.4×10^{-2}	1.3×10^{-1}
Sr	21	3.4×10^{-2}	3.2×10^{-2}	2.6×10^{-2}	2.1	9.3×10^{-3}	1.3×10^{-1}
Te	1	1.3×10^{-2}					
U	1	4.8×10^{-4}					
Zr	1	1.7×10^{-5}					

N Sample size, *AM* arithmetic mean, *ASD* arithmetic standard deviation, *GM* geometric mean, *GSD* geometric standard deviation,
Howard et al. (2016a, b)
*The mean is a geometric mean except where the number of data values (N) is less than 3, in which case it is a n arithmetic mean. Further statistical information is given for a wider range of radionuclides in TECDOC 1616 and TRS 472 (IAEA 2009, 2010)

5.4.2.1 Radioiodine

The deposition of atmospheric iodine (mainly from marine sources) onto the aerial parts of plants is an important contributor to stable iodine (^{127}I) in plants and is a major source for grazing animals. Iodine intake by agricultural animals is also enhanced by consumption of cattle feed fortified with iodine and the use of iodine-containing sterilants in the dairy industry.

Unlike many of the other radionuclides that affect the food chain, stable iodine is essential for normal growth and development in animals (including humans). It accumulates in various organs and tissues of the body, notably the thyroid. The major function of the thyroid gland is to produce the thyroid hormones, T4 (thyroxine) and the more active T3 (triiodothyronine), so it accumulates iodine from the plasma to produce these compounds.

Raw milk is one of the foods that are most likely rapidly to become contaminated by radioiodine as livestock feeds on grass which has been contaminated by deposited radioiodine. Radioiodine isotopes intercepted by pasture vegetation ingested by grazing animals such as dairy cows, goats and sheep are quickly and completely absorbed through the gut (Howard et al. 1996a, b; Vandecasteele et al. 2000). The consumption of different physico-chemical forms of iodine does not change the extent of true absorption which is consistently complete (i.e. F_a is 1) (Howard et al. 1996a, b; Vandecasteele et al. 2000). Furthermore, there is no reduction in gut absorption of radioiodine isotopes due to enhanced stable iodine intake. Iodine is rapidly absorbed into the blood plasma where it circulates as an iodide and from which it is subsequently accumulated in the thyroid. Radioiodine is also transferred into the mammary gland and excreted via milk. It is also excreted via urine.

The capacity of the thyroid to concentrate iodine magnifies the hazard imposed by ^{131}I as it is accumulated in a similar manner to stable iodine. Therefore, it accumulates in the thyroid and also rapidly transfers into the milk within 30 min of introduction into the body (Thorell 1964). Peak radioiodine activity concentrations will be reached in 6–12 h. Radioactive iodine can also be absorbed via the lung into the plasma.

Goat's milk and sheep's milk contain approximately tenfold higher radioiodine activity concentration than cow's milk. For cows the milk/plasma ratio has been reported as 0.6–5.5, whereas for sheep and goats, it was 2–24 (Lengemann 1970).

In a controlled feeding experiment, using herbage recently contaminated by fallout from the Chernobyl NRE, the transfer coefficient of ^{131}I to sheep milk was 0.3 ± 0.017 d/L (Howard et al. 1993). These data are similar to F_m values reported for iodine for sheep milk in TRS 472 (IAEA 2010) of 0.23 d/L (geometric mean) and varied from 0.03 to 0.9 d/L. Similar values of F_m (range 0.015–0.020 d/L) after the Chernobyl NRE were reported for stable iodine in dairy cows by Vandecasteele et al. (2000). The daily proportion of ^{131}I intake which was secreted in sheep milk was $5.6 \pm 0.035\%$ which is an order of magnitude higher than for cattle and agrees with the higher transfer of stable iodine from plasma to milk which occurs in sheep and goats. The lactation phase does not seem to have a significant effect on iodine transfer to milk (Vandecasteele et al. 2000).

As for humans, it is important to establish the effect of stable iodine intake for dairy animals. In controlled experiments, Vandecasteele et al. (2000) reported that the mean F_m values for oral radioiodine to milk increased from 0.020 d/L for a low stable iodine intake to 0.024 d/L for a moderate stable iodine rate. There was a significant decrease in the transfer to milk for the high stable dietary iodine intake rate (mean F_m of 0.018 d/L) compared with the moderate treatment. The differences for the three stable iodine treatments were due to differential affinities and saturation levels of the thyroid and milk pathways competing for the available iodine.

Associated modelling studies confirmed that the stable iodine intake may affect the partitioning of iodine between thyroid, milk and excreta (Crout et al. 2000). The model was used to predict the effects of variation in stable iodine intake and the extent of consequent chemical contamination of milk by stable iodine. The predicted time taken for radioiodine to reach peak concentrations in milk following a deposition event varied significantly (ca. 2 days) over a range of stable iodine intakes. Administration of low amounts of stable iodine of <100 mg/d to dairy animals could increase F_m, whereas >150 mg/d stable iodine would reduce radioiodine transfer to milk. However, administration of sufficient stable iodine to reduce the radioiodine transfer to milk would result in stable iodine concentrations in milk that were greatly in excess of internationally advised limits. Therefore, increased stable iodine supplementation should not be used as a countermeasure to reduce radioiodine transfer to milk due to the elevated stable iodine in milk (Howard et al. 1996a, b).

The $T_{1/2}^{b}$ of ^{131}I measured in ewes that were moved from contaminated pasture to housing and then fed an ^{131}I-free diet was 1 day, accounting for 97.4% of the reduction in the ^{131}I activity concentration in milk. Data on $T_{1/2}^{b}$ in cow, goat and sheep milk show consistently fast reduction at 1–2 days (Howard et al. 1993; Fesenko et al. 2015), and it is longer in various organs, e.g. thyroid, 100 days; bone, 14 days; and kidney, spleen and reproductive organs, 7 days.

Radioiodine in milk was an important contributor to internal dose in the emergency response phase and the initial part of the transition phase after the Chernobyl NRE. The ingested radioiodine was completely absorbed in the gut and rapidly transferred to the animals' thyroid and milk (within about 1 day). Throughout the contaminated areas of the USSR and parts of Eastern and Western Europe, peak ^{131}I activity concentrations in milk occurred rapidly after deposition in late April or early May 1986 depending on when the radioactive contamination reached each county. Therefore, transfer of ^{131}I to milk was the initial priority.

The ^{131}I activity concentration in milk after the Chernobyl NRE decreased with an $T_{1/2}^{eff}$ of 4–5 days due to its short physical half-life and the reduction in iodine activity concentrations on plants due to various removal processes from leaf surfaces. The removal rate, measured as a mean weathering half-life on grass, was about 9 days for radioiodine and 11 days for radiocaesium (Kirchner 1994).

5.4.2.2 Radiocaesium

Radiocaesium can be ingested or inhaled. The most important isotope with a physical half-life of 30 years is ^{137}Cs. Cs-134 has a shorter physical half-life of ~2 years, so its relative importance declines much faster than that of ^{137}Cs.

After the Chernobyl NRE, from June 1986, radiocaesium was the dominant radionuclide in most environmental samples and in food products contributing to the human food chain. The contamination of milk with radiocaesium decreased during spring 1986 with an $T_{1/2}^{eff}$ of about 2 weeks due to weathering, biomass growth and other natural processes. The amount and type of feed ingested by dairy cattle changes considerably during the course of lactation and with season leading to temporal variations in radiocaesium transfer to milk. Radiocaesium activity concentrations increased in many countries during winter 1986/1987 due to cows being fed with contaminated hay harvested in spring/summer 1986.

The physical and chemical form in which radiocaesium is ingested substantially affects the extent of absorption across the gut and the subsequent radiocaesium activity concentrations in animals and animal products. Radiocaesium absorption varies over a 50-fold range, depending upon dietary source (Beresford et al. 2000). Radiocaesium recently deposited after the Chernobyl NRE onto leaf surfaces was initially less available for gut absorption (F_a of 0.24) than that when it was plant-incorporated (Howard et al. 1989; Beresford et al. 2000). Once radiocaesium is incorporated into the internal plant structure through leaf absorption or root uptake, it is more highly absorbed in the GI tract (F_a of 0.8–1.0). The absorption of sediment- or soil-associated radiocaesium may be lower than that in plant-incorporated form and will vary for different types of soil (as does plant uptake) (Beresford et al. 2000). The availability for biological uptake of radionuclides associated with fuel particles that were deposited mostly within a 50 km radius of the Chernobyl NPP was lower than for plant-incorporated sources.

There were differing rates of ^{137}Cs transfer to milk in areas with different soil types. The transfer to milk declines in the order as follows: peat bog > sandy and sandy loam > chernozem and grey forest soils.

The $T_{1/2}^{b}$ of radiocaesium in milk is fast at 1–2 days (Fesenko et al. 2015) so the ^{137}Cs or ^{134}Cs activity concentrations in milk from dairy cows removed from contaminated areas declined rapidly. The long-term time trend of radiocaesium activity concentrations in milk (and meat) roughly follows that for vegetation (with a time lag) and can be divided into two time periods (Fesenko et al. 1997). For the first 4–6 years after deposition of Chernobyl NRE radiocaesium, there was an initial fast decrease with an ecological half-life between 0.8 and 1.2 years. Later, the rate of decline was slower and varied with soil type (Fesenko et al. 1997).

5.4.2.3 Radiostrontium

The behaviour of strontium in all organisms is strongly influenced by the presence of its analogue, calcium. The calcium requirement of an animal varies due to factors such as milk yield and stage of pregnancy (Howard et al. 1997). In response to these requirements, the calcium intake of dairy animals changes throughout the year. Typically, the calcium intake by dairy goats will range from 15 to 30 g/d, whilst that of cows will be 70–150 g/d (Beresford et al. 1998).

The gastrointestinal absorption of radiostrontium is less dependent upon dietary source than that of radiocaesium. Calcium status is generally the controlling influence on strontium absorption. The absorption of calcium is homeostatically controlled, and the extent of absorption is determined by animals' requirement for growth, milk production, etc. When calcium intake is in excess of requirement than for all sources, the F_a for Sr is 0.1–0.3. For a given calcium requirement, Ca absorption is inversely proportional to dietary Ca intake. Hence, Sr absorption should also be inversely proportional (Comar 1966). Collated data from experiments after the Kyshtym NRE, which included a number of data with relatively low ratios of calcium intake to requirement, and other data reported during the period of global weapons fallout, showed a clear reduction in the F_m of ^{90}Sr with an increasing ratio of intake/requirement for calcium (Beresford et al. 1998).

The use of the reported mean F_m for radiostrontium in Howard et al. (2016b, 2017) is only appropriate for productive agricultural systems where calcium is readily available (Comar 1966; Howard et al. 1997). F_m may be higher in low-productivity regions with low calcium intakes.

The $T^b_{1/2}$ of ^{90}Sr in milk is fast at 1–2 days (Fesenko et al. 2015), so the ^{90}Sr activity concentrations in milk from dairy cows that are removed from contaminated areas will decline rapidly.

5.4.3 *Meat and Offal Production*

Different radionuclides are accumulated in different tissues. The most important tissue for the food chain of many countries is muscle for which the data is much more extensive than that for other accumulating tissues.

5.4.3.1 Transfer of Radionuclides to Meat

Within a few weeks of the Chernobyl NRE, there were high reported ^{137}Cs and ^{134}Cs activity concentrations in the muscle of ruminants, resulting in intensive monitoring of meat from cattle, goats, sheep, reindeer, game and fish. Data on the transfer of radiocaesium to different animals has been reported from many countries after the Chernobyl NRE; there are much more data available for cow meat than for any other agricultural animal. The transfer of radiocaesium to meat is higher than that to milk. The extent of transfer of radionuclides into the meat of different types of animals is given as both F_f and CR values in TRS 472; selected relevant values for F_f are shown in Tables 5.14, 5.15, 5.16, 5.17 and 5.18 and for CR in Table 5.19.

Table 5.14 Transfer coefficients for radionuclides relevant for NREs to cow meat d/kg

Element	N	Reference value	Minimum	Maximum
Am	1	5.0×10^{-4}		
Co	4	4.3×10^{-4}	1.3×10^{-4}	8.4×10^{-4}
Cs	58	2.2×10^{-2}	4.7×10^{-3}	9.6×10^{-2}
I	5	6.7×10^{-3}	2.0×10^{-3}	3.8×10^{-2}
Nb	1	2.6×10^{-7}		
Pu	5	1.1×10^{-6}	8.8×10^{-8}	3.0×10^{-4}
Ru	3	3.3×10^{-3}	2.2×10^{-3}	6.4×10^{-3}
Sr	35	1.3×10^{-3}	2.0×10^{-4}	9.2×10^{-3}
Te	1	7.0×10^{-3}		
U	3	3.9×10^{-4}	2.5×10^{-4}	6.3×10^{-4}
Zr	1	1.2×10^{-6}		

IAEA (2010)

Table 5.15 Transfer coefficients for radionuclides relevant for NREs to sheep meat d/kg

Element	N	Reference value	Minimum	Maximum
Ag	1	4.8×10^{-4}		
Am	1	1.1×10^{-4}		
Ce	1	2.5×10^{-4}		
Co	2	1.2×10^{-2}	8.0×10^{-3}	1.6×10^{-2}
Cs	41	1.9×10^{-1}	5.3×10^{-2}	1.3
I	1	3.0×10^{-2}		
Pu	2	5.3×10^{-5}	2.0×10^{-5}	8.5×10^{-5}
Ru	2	2.1×10^{-3}	6.3×10^{-4}	3.6×10^{-3}
S	3	1.7	1.2	2.1
Sr	25	1.5×10^{-3}	3.0×10^{-4}	4.0×10^{-3}

IAEA (2010)

Table 5.16 Transfer coefficients for radionuclides relevant for NREs to goat meat d/kg

Element	N	Reference value	Minimum	Maximum
Cs	11	3.2×10^{-1}	1.2×10^{-1}	1.9
Nb	1	6.0×10^{-5}		
Sr	8	2.9×10^{-3}	2.0×10^{-3}	3.7×10^{-3}
Te	1	2.4×10^{-3}		
Zr	1	2.0×10^{-5}		

IAEA (2010)

Table 5.17 Transfer coefficients for radionuclides relevant for NREs to pig meat d/kg

Element	N	Reference value	Minimum	Maximum
Cs	22	2.0×10^{-1}	1.2×10^{-1}	4.0×10^{-1}
I	2	4.1×10^{-2}	1.5×10^{-2}	6.6×10^{-2}
Ru	1	3.0×10^{-3}		
Sr	12	2.5×10^{-3}	5.0×10^{-4}	8.0×10^{-3}
U	2	4.4×10^{-2}	2.6×10^{-2}	6.2×10^{-2}

IAEA (2010)

Table 5.18 Transfer coefficients for radionuclides relevant for NREs to poultry meat d/kg

Element	N	Reference value	Minimum	Maximum
Co	2	9.7×10^{-1}	3.0×10^{-2}	1.9
Cs	13	2.7	1.2	5.6
I	3	8.7×10^{-3}	4.0×10^{-3}	1.5×10^{-2}
Nb	1	3.0×10^{-4}		
Po	1	2.4		
Sr	7	2.0×10^{-2}	7.0×10^{-3}	4.1×10^{-2}
Te	1	6.0×10^{-1}		
U	2	7.5×10^{-1}	3.0×10^{-1}	1.2
Zr	1	6.0×10^{-5}		

IAEA (2010)

Table 5.19 Concentration ratios for radionuclides relevant for NREs to the meat of different animals

	Cattle				Sheep				Pork				Generic
Element	CR	Minimum	Maximum	N	CR	Minimum	Maximum	N	CR	Minimum	Maximum	N	
Ag					4.3×10^{-4}			1					4.3×10^{-4}
Am					1.1×10^{-4}			1					1.1×10^{-4}
Ce					2.2×10^{-4}			1					2.2×10^{-4}
Co	3.9×10^{-1}	7.2×10^{-3}	7.8×10^{-1}	2	2.3×10^{-1}								3.1×10^{-1}
Cs	2.3×10^{-1}	2.2×10^{-2}	7.3×10^{-1}	17	6.4×10^{-1}	5.3×10^{-2}	7.5	51	9.2×10^{-2}	8.3×10^{-3}	2.4×10^{-1}	4	3.9×10^{-1}[a]
I	9.5×10^{-2}	3.2×10^{-2}	1.9×10^{-1}	3				1	9.3×10^{-2}	3.5×10^{-2}	1.5×10^{-1}	2	9.4×10^{-2}
Nb	6.5×10^{-6}			1									6.5×10^{-6}
Po	1.4×10^{-1}	3.7×10^{-2}	4.1×10^{-1}	7									1.4×10^{-1}
Pu					3.9×10^{-5}	1.5×10^{-5}	6.3×10^{-5}	3					3.9×10^{-5}
Ru					5.7×10^{-4}			1					5.7×10^{-4}
S					5.0×10^{-1}								5.0×10^{-1}
Te	1.8×10^{-1}			1									1.8×10^{-1}
U	3.3×10^{-1}	3.0×10^{-3}	1.7	8									3.3×10^{-1}
Zn	1.7	4.7×10^{-1}	3.2	9	2.1	1.3	2.9	2					1.9

[a]Goat value of 6.2×10^{-1} for Cs (n = 4) is included in the generic value

IAEA (2010)

5.4.3.2 Other Accumulating Tissues

The transfer of radionuclides to eggs is high compared with meat. Transfer parameter values for eggs are listed in Table 5.20 and are largely based on data from chickens. There are F_f values reported by a number of sources for the three key elements, I, Cs and Sr, but few values for most other elements.

5.4.3.3 Target Tissues for Different Radionuclides

Some radionuclides accumulate in specific organs. The key accumulating organs in animals for radionuclides released during NREs is shown in Table 5.21. The table is largely based on a review of Russian language literature which reported F_f values

Table 5.20 Transfer coefficients for radionuclides relevant for NREs to egg contents d/kg

Element	N	GM	Minimum	Maximum
Am	1	3.0×10^{-3}		
Ce	1	3.1×10^{-3}		
Co	2	3.3×10^{-2}	2.6×10^{-2}	4.0×10^{-2}
Cs	11	4.0×10^{-1}	1.6×10^{-1}	7.1×10^{-1}
I	4	2.4	1.9	3.2
Nb	1	1.0×10^{-3}		
Po	1	3.1		
Pu	2	1.2×10^{-3}	9.9 × 10–6	2.3×10^{-3}
Ru	1	4.0×10^{-3}		
Sr	9	4.9×10^{-1}	2.5×10^{-1}	4.8
Te	1	5.1		
U	2	1.1	9.2×10^{-1}	1.2
Zr	1	2.0×10^{-4}		

IAEA (2010)

Table 5.21 Accumulating organs for different radionuclides

Radionuclide	Accumulating organs
Ag	Liver
Am	Bone and liver
Ce	Bone, kidney and liver
Co	Liver and kidney
Cs	All soft tissue except adipose tissue
I	Thyroid and milk
Pu	Bone and liver
Ru	Kidney and liver
Sb	Liver
Sr	Bone
Tc	Thyroid, liver and stomach wall

Fesenko et al. (2018)

for various organs consumed by humans (Fesenko et al. 2018). Radiocaesium is present at similar activity concentration in most soft tissue (and tends to be higher in the kidney, but not consistently) with lower accumulation in bone and adipose tissue. Many heavy metal radionuclides accumulate in the liver. No relevant transfer parameter data for ^{210}Po or ^{95}Zr have been identified.

5.5 Radionuclide Transfer in Non-intensive Animal Production

The Chernobyl fallout contaminated large areas of the terrestrial environment with a major impact on animal production on unimproved land. Depending on the weather patterns for the first 2 weeks after the NRE, parts of Eastern and Western Europe were contaminated, especially where the passage of the contaminated fall-out in the atmosphere coincided with heavy rainfall. These areas included upland areas and clearings within, or bordering woodland. They are collectively termed here as non-intensive systems (but also called seminatural, extensive systems or free-ranging systems). In these areas, unfertilized, highly organic soils are often used for extensive agricultural production of animal products, mainly for grazing by ruminants, such as sheep, goats, reindeer and cattle, on alpine meadows and upland regions. Therefore, problems with animal products were widely experienced not only within the USSR but also in many other countries in Europe.

The initial impact of radionuclide deposition on these systems, as for intensive systems, depended on the extent of interception by plants consumed by the animals. Thereafter, soil to plant to animal transfer dominated. These systems are potentially important after NREs due to the prevailing soil types and vegetation species which can allow relatively higher, and more prolonged, radiocaesium transfer to animals compared with intensively managed agricultural production (Howard et al. 1991, 1996a, b).

Normal agricultural practices which often reduced the transfer of radionuclides from soils to plant by physical dilution (e.g. ploughing) or by adding competitive elements (e.g. fertilizing) are generally not applied in these systems due to the low depth of soil and presence of stones and rocks. The low potassium status and high organic matter content of the soil in these often-unfertilized areas enhance the movement of radiocaesium from soil constituents into the soil solution from which it can be taken up by plants.

After the Chernobyl NRE, the high radiocaesium uptake from peaty soil in unmanaged (termed extensive) grassland was particularly important for a number of European countries where such land was used for the grazing of ruminants and the production of hay. Contamination with radiocaesium in animal food products from these radioecologically sensitive, non-intensive ecosystems often persisted for decades, even though the original deposition may not have been high (Howard et al. 2002). This is largely because there was prolonged and significant plant uptake of radiocaesium from soil and some plant and other species consumed by animals accumulated high levels of radiocaesium, such as ericaceous species (e.g. heather) and mushrooms.

Animals kept on unimproved land had higher radiocaesium activity concentrations than those from agricultural systems after both the Chernobyl and Fukushima Daiichi NREs. Little information is available for other radionuclides and there is no current evidence of significant long-term problems with other radionuclides in these production systems.

5.5.1 Dairy Production in Low-Productivity Areas

In some countries, such as Austria and Norway, non-intensive systems are used during the growing season for dairy animals where suitable upland pastures exist and there are adequate facilities to carry out milking within a suitable distance. Some of these mountainous regions of Western European countries were amongst the most contaminated territories outside of the former USSR after the Chernobyl NRE. In these non-intensive systems, vertical migration rate of ^{137}Cs is slow, so it remains in the upper soil layer where root uptake of nutrients often occurs. A relatively high radiocaesium soil-to-vegetation transfer was reported in some of these pastures (e.g. Norway). Activity concentration of ^{137}Cs in milk in such areas rose quickly in the first 2 weeks after the dairy animals began to graze these regions (around mid-June) and remained elevated until the animals were removed in the autumn. Activity concentrations of ^{137}Cs in milk on such meadows during summertime were several orders of magnitude higher than in milk from lowland areas and valleys, where intensive agriculture occurs (IAEA 1994; Lettner et al. 2007). The ^{137}Cs activity concentration of milk would have remained above the intervention levels for many years if remediation options had not been applied. For example, ^{137}Cs activity concentrations in milk from Austrian sites remained high even 17 years after the Chernobyl NRE reflecting the persistent elevated transfer of radiocaesium from poorer soils in alpine pastures and regions with silicate bedrock.

Considerably longer ecological half-lives have been observed in cow's milk from alpine pastures than in cow's milk from lowland production sites. For the period 1988–2006, Lettner et al. (2007)) derived ecological half-lives of 0.7–1.4 years for the fast loss component and of 9.3–12.7 years for the slow loss component of ^{137}Cs activity concentrations in cow's milk. Later studies showed that the $T_{1/2}^{eff}$ and mean altitude of the alpine meadows sites were positively correlated, with higher altitude sites having significantly longer half-lives than those at lower altitudes. Depending on the site, half-lives varied from about 4 and 15 years (Lettner et al. 2009).

5.5.2 *Meat Production in Low-Productivity Areas*

After the Chernobyl NPP, the transfer of radiocaesium to meat of grazing stock in non-intensive areas was also higher than that in lowland regions in several countries, including Norway and the United Kingdom due to the same factors discussed for dairy animals. Free-ranging stock that graze these areas include sheep, cattle and goats; such land is also used for rearing game animals such as grouse, pheasant and partridge.

There was considerable variation in radiocaesium activity concentrations between individual animals within the same grazing areas. Reasons for the variation included individual preferences in the areas being grazed as there was considerable spatial variation on the deposition density of radiocaesium, even within a few metres, and the range of different vegetation species present.

Metabolic variation was also important. For example, there was considerable variability in the radiocaesium activity concentration of muscle between individual sheep in the same free ranging flock in contaminated upland areas of the United Kingdom (Beresford et al. 1996). Certain sheep within a flock were consistently amongst the most contaminated, whereas others were consistently the least contaminated (Beresford et al. 1995; Walters 1988). When ionic radiocaesium was orally administered to 22 sheep under controlled conditions, the F_f varied by three-fold. The $T^b_{1/2}$ in muscle varied from 5 to 19 days with a mean of 9.8 days. Changes in live weight and feed intake during the study together accounted for 72% of the variation in the F_f values, and live weight change accounted for 56% of the observed variation in biological half-life. The data suggested that variation in metabolism of radiocaesium contributes to the variability in radiocaesium activity concentrations within sheep flocks in areas contaminated by Chernobyl fallout.

Contaminated animals raised for meat production cannot be sampled as easily as the milk from dairy animals. The development of equipment that was suitable for live monitoring of animals *in situ* in these areas was important in managing the situation and developing suitable remediation strategies.

5.6 Radionuclide Transfer to Game Animals

5.6.1 *Forest Environments*

The primary concern regarding forests from a radiological perspective is the long-term contamination of the forest environment and its products with ^{137}Cs due to its 30-year half-life. However, ^{134}Cs should not be forgotten as it may be present in large quantities and can significantly contribute to the contamination of animal products for more than a decade. The meat of game animals grazing in contaminated forests often has high radiocaesium activity concentrations.

Other radionuclides in forests such as the plutonium isotopes are of limited significance for animal products due to their low environmental mobility.

Substantial radioactive contamination of forests occurred following the Chernobyl and Fukushima Daiichi NREs. The deposition density of ^{137}Cs in Ukraine, Belarus and Russia exceeded >10 MBq/m^2 in some forested areas. In several Western European countries, such as Finland, Sweden, Norway, Germany and Austria, the deposition density of ^{137}Cs was also relatively high compared to other sources such as global fallout. After the Fukushima NRE, the extensive forest catchments in Fukushima prefecture covered about 70% of the most contaminated areas.

In many of the affected countries, the extent of game meat consumption from seminatural areas and forests by the general population was low compared with agricultural animal products. However, there were specific groups such as hunters who may consume relatively large quantities of game meat. Tree canopies, particularly at forest edges, are efficient filters of atmospheric pollutants of all kinds. The primary mechanism of tree contamination after the NREs was direct interception of radiocaesium of between 60 and 90% of the initial deposition by the tree canopy (Tikhomirov et al. 1994; Kato et al. 2012). Radionuclides on tree surfaces were gradually transferred to the upper layers of soil through natural weathering and wash-off by rainwater. Within a few years after deposition, most of the radiocaesium was transferred from the tree canopy to the underlying soil which became the major repository of radiocaesium contamination within the forest. The upper soil layers acted as a long-term sink and source of radiocaesium contamination of forest vegetation and animals.

A wide range of plants and fungi are consumed by wild animals in forests. Higher transfer of radiocaesium occurred from soil to some plants including grasses, lichens and berries, and also to mushrooms and truffles. Individual plant and fungal species differed greatly in their ability to accumulate radiocaesium, with particularly high radiocaesium activity concentrations in some mushroom species (IAEA 2010). The high levels of contamination in various mushroom species are reflected in generally high soil-mushroom Tag values which can vary by a factor of about 2000 (IAEA 2009, 2010).

Contamination of mushrooms in forests is often much higher than that of forest fruits such as bilberries. The Tag values for forest berries range from 0.02 to 0.2 m^2/kg (IAEA 2009, 2010).

The shooting of game animals or snaring of other species is often, but not always, confined to certain seasons, so the short-term impact of radionuclide deposition can initially be highly dependent on when the NRE occurs relative to the shooting season. After the transition phase, the spatial and temporal variability in contamination of game animals is affected by many different factors including:

- Highly heterogeneous deposition of radionuclides onto forests and associated terrain
- Spatial variation in soil type and therefore soil to plant transfer of radiocaesium
- Vertical migration of radiocaesium down the soil profile and out of the rooting zone
- Forest-specific differences in available edible food sources
- Seasonal variations in diet composition and feeding behaviour of game species

- Consumption of highly contaminated mushrooms and truffles
- The number of days with a heavy snow cover or ice
- $T_{1/2}^{b}$ which is longer on larger species such as moose/elk
- $T_{1/2}^{eff}$ which varies with time, species and forest characteristics

Significant variations occur in the body burden of radiocaesium in game animals due to the seasonal availability of the various components of their diet (IAEA 2009). Species-specific information on how the above factors affect some of the main species affected by radiocaesium deposition is provided in Table 5.22.

Table 5.22 General trends for radiocaesium in forest animals

Game animal	Diet	Seasonal trend in radiocaesium activity concentrations in meat
Roe deer, white-tailed deer	Winter–summer – wide variety of herbs and grasses, leaf buds and small twigs of trees and shrub Autumn – also mushrooms, lichen	Autumn peak associated with mushroom consumption
Red deer	Fibre-rich diet. Do not consume mushrooms	Not evident
Wild boar	Omnivorous diet that varies considerably with season Spring and summer – mostly herbivorous, plants Autumn – mushrooms Winter – often burrow into soil and feed on roots, tubers, larvae and earthworms and truffles with more radiocaesium than green plants; also consuming contaminated soil when burrowing. Consumption of beechnuts and acorns can reduce radiocaesium intake	The seasonal change in diet, combined with mushroom consumption during autumn and winter, can lead to an up to twofold increase in winter than in the spring and summer. However, diet intake can be highly variable in the different seasons, increasing with mushroom, truffle and soil consumption
Moose or elk	Herbivore – consumes many types of terrestrial vegetation, mainly consisting of forbs and other non-grasses, and fresh shoots from trees such as willow and birch. Therefore, soil type is a key variable	Higher in winter than in summer when moose often have access to pastures
Reindeer and caribou	Summer – a wide range of plants Autumn – consumption of mushrooms increases the radiocaesium intake Winter – consumption of lichens, which retain a high proportion of deposited radiocaesium and have a low K content. The change in diet is accompanied by a two- to threefold increase in the biological half-life of radiocaesium from about 7 to about 20 days	Highest in winter During summer and early autumn, only 10–20% (or less) of that in winter Higher in autumn than in the summer

Based on Skuterud et al. (2004), Strebl and Tataruch (2007), IAEA (2009, 2010)

Table 5.23 Comparison of Tag values for game animals obtained within 5 years after the Fukushima Daiichi and Chernobyl NREs

Species or group	Range of GM Tag values (m^2/kg fm)	
	Fukushima NRE (Tagami et al. 2016)	Chernobyl NRE (IAEA 2009)
Deer	$5.1 \times 10^{-3} - 7.2 \times 10^{-3}$	$7.6 \times 10^{-3} - 9.4 \times 10^{-2}$ $2.8 \times 10^{-2} - 5.0 \times 10^{-2}$
Wild boar	$2.6 \times 10^{-3} - 6.8 \times 10^{-3}$	$4.0 \times 10^{-3} - 6.7 \times 10^{-2}$
Bear	$2.8 \times 10^{-3} - 5.2 \times 10^{-3}$	$4.3 \times 10^{-2} - 7.1 \times 10^{-2}$
Pheasant	$1.6 \times 10^{-3} - 4.8 \times 10^{-3}$ $1.0 \times 10^{-4} - 8.9 \times 10^{-4}$	3.2×10^{-4}
Wild duck	$2.2 \times 10^{-4} - 8.7 \times 10^{-4}$	$2.4 \times 10^{-3} - 1.3 \times 10^{-2}$

Tagami et al. (2016), IAEA (2009)

Tag values have been reported in numerous publications, but it is difficult to identify generally applicable trends due to the wide variation in spatial and temporal trends. Tag values are often higher for wild boar than other species and the difference seems to increase with time. Also Tag values for the larger ruminants such as red deer and moose are often lower than for small deer and wild boar. Tag values compiled for the first 5 years after the Fukushima Daiichi accident, for three species, are compared with the equivalent period for Chernobyl NRE in Table 5.23.

Since the NREs, the natural decontamination of forest plants and, therefore, animals has been much slower than that in agricultural areas. Wild ruminants with access to agricultural land often have lower radiocaesium concentrations than those grazing inside forests (Kiefer et al. 1996).

The prevailing conditions in many forests, with often low potassium contents and high organic matter contents in the upper soil layers, and consequently high uptake of radiocaesium by some plants and mushrooms, lead to long $T_{1/2}^{eff}$ of radiocaesium in game animals. After the Chernobyl NRE, the $T_{1/2}^{eff}$ of ^{137}Cs in game meat varied from about 3 to 10 years. Over several decades, the physical decay rate of ^{137}Cs has been the key factor determining the rate of reduction in ^{137}Cs activity concentrations in some forest game animals.

5.7 Impacts on the Health of Livestock Exposed to Nuclear Contamination

A key feature of both the Kyshtym and Chernobyl NREs was the difference in the impact on the health of livestock between the emergency response phase, when there was an initial, intensive short-term radiation impact, and the subsequent transition phase, with a slow decline in the dose rate. Doses from radioactivity that may endanger the health and well-being of livestock are only likely to occur in the immediate vicinity of a major NRE involving a nuclear reactor.

To reliably estimate the impact of post-NRE doses to farm animals, information needs to be collected soon after the NRE for animals remaining in these areas. The limited data available for the period after NRE have been reviewed by Fesenko (2019) for the Kyshtym NRE and Geras'kin et al. (2008) and other sources given below who focused on the Chernobyl NRE.

The exposure routes for animals remaining in areas that have been highly contaminated include:

- External exposure from highly contaminated surfaces such as contaminated soil and surfaces of trees
- Internal exposure from consumption of highly contaminated plant material leading to direct irradiation of the digestive tract
- Internal exposure due to the absorption of radionuclides through the gut and accumulation into the tissues

There are considerable challenges associated with collecting relevant data for agricultural animals after a NRE. It is difficult to accurately estimate the doses received which vary greatly with location and with time. Some problems experienced after the Chernobyl NRE given by Geras'kin et al. (2008) include:

- Extreme small- and large-scale heterogeneity in the extent of radioactive contamination in affected areas due to the prolonged period of intensive radionuclide releases and variable meteorological conditions, combined with the wide spectrum of deposited radionuclides.
- High uncertainty in the estimation of doses received for observed biological effects. In the emergency response phase, radiation monitoring will inevitably be insufficient to allow a robust, reliable estimation of the consequent biological effects. Rapid changes of doses to agricultural animals occur due to the decay of short-lived radionuclides, radionuclide redistribution in the environment, changes in contribution of different radionuclides to different exposure pathways and the presence of highly contaminated particles.
- Difficulty in estimation of radiation effects due to the lack of verified methods for reconstruction of absorbed doses to living organisms in the complex emergency response phase.
- Changes in the sensitivity of animals to radiation doses during the different stages of growth, which can vary by orders of magnitude.

Dose Estimation After the Kyshtym NRE Information from the Kyshtym NRE is summarized here based on a recent review by Fesenko (2019). In contrast to the Chernobyl NRE, the Kyshtym NRE did not release short-lived radioiodine isotopes. Domesticated cattle and sheep were the most exposed agricultural animals after the Kyshtym NRE with initial radiation effects for domesticated animals being observed shortly after the NRE. The decision to evacuate both the public and animals living in the most affected areas was taken 12 days after the NRE. During that time the animals were grazing pasture with a total contamination density (combining all radionuclides released) of around 900-1000 MBq m^{-2} and received estimated external doses of 1.4–3.0 Gy. The corresponding doses to the GI tract were higher and reached 4–24 Gy. The radiation doses resulted in a high mortality rate of exposed cattle with symptoms that could be attributed to acute radiation sickness, including bleeding of mucous membranes and leucopoenia.

The cattle grazing slightly further away from the most contaminated area received lower external doses of about 0.1 Gy and doses to the GI tract of 1.0–2.0 Gy. These animals survived although some detrimental changes occurred in the blood-producing metabolic systems that produce blood components over the first 6 months.

Similar effects were observed for highly contaminated sheep. Sheep grazing on sites close to the source of the release received external doses of 1.4–3 Gy and absorbed doses to the GI tract of 8–54 Gy during the first 12 days after the NRE and before evacuation. As for the cattle, the doses caused symptoms of acute radiation sickness and death in most of the animals.

No substantial radiation effects were observed in sheep at less contaminated sites (100–200 MBq m^{-2} of total radioactivity). For these sheep, the calculated doses during the first 12 days after the NRE were 0.1–0.2 Gy, and the GI tract doses were 2–4 Gy. Over the next few months, temporary changes in the blood-producing system of these animals occurred after evacuation.

An absorbed dose of around 1 Gy to the GI tract of large herbivores led to a reduction in wild game populations. Some reduction in the number of moose and roe deer occurred in 1957–1958 in areas where the GI tract doses would have been 10–30 Gy. However, increased mortality of large animals was not documented due to the difficulty in locating animals. At sites with a lower ^{90}Sr deposition density of 37 MBq m^{-2}, animals could have received an additional external dose of 2–3 Gy. At such doses, early radiation effects and even death of some animals may have occurred.

Dose Estimation After the Chernobyl NRE Appraisals of the effects of radiation on livestock inhabiting the area immediately surrounding the nuclear power plant at Chernobyl have been reported in the last decade (Fesenko et al. 2005; Geras'kin et al. 2008). Initially, there was an acute phase of radiation exposure of approximately 3–4 weeks that was due to the short-lived radionuclides, including ^{131}I deposited on vegetation and the ground surface. High exposure of the thyroids of vertebrates occurred due to inhalation and ingestion of radioiodine isotopes. Approximately 80% of the total radiation dose accumulated by animals were received within the first three months after the NRE, mostly due to ß-radiation. A second phase of exposure followed in the autumn of 1986 when the short-lived radionuclides had decayed, due to environmental pathways that transported various longer-lived radionuclides. The third stage of radiation exposure, continuing to the present day, is chronic exposure due mainly to ^{137}Cs.

A review of radiation doses and effects by Geras'kin et al. (2008) for the Chernobyl NRE has been used as the source of much of the information summarized here. The large-scale and heterogeneous radioactive contamination of the affected areas led to a variety of responses at different levels of molecular and cellular biological organization. The most affected livestock were within the 30 km

Chernobyl NPP zone when the highest exposures occurred during the first 10–20 days after the NRE. The major contributors to the absorbed dose in this period were short-lived radionuclides.

Radiation damage to agricultural animals was largely caused by the accumulation of various radioiodine isotopes in the thyroid. In the first 240 days after the NRE, the ratio of absorbed doses from all sources of exposure between the thyroid, GI tract mucosa and whole body was 230:1.2:1 (Alexakhin et al. 1992).

Doses received by farm animals depended on the deposition density of radionuclides at their locations and their residence time in the contaminated regions. Doses to the GI tract mucosa in a few cattle grazing in the 30 km zone reached 10 Gy over the first month after the NRE. The doses were about 7 Gy to tens of thousands of evacuated animals and about 1 Gy in the remaining livestock (Alexakhin et al. 2004). There was a 69% and 82% reduction in thyroid function in cattle associated with an estimated thyroid dose of 50 Gy and 280 Gy, respectively (Astasheva et al. 1991).

Animals that remained in the exclusion zone for several months had impaired immune responses, lowered body temperatures and cardiovascular disorders. Increased lethality was observed in evacuated cows 5–8 months after the NRE. Damage included partial atrophy or total destruction of the thyroid, liver degeneration, increased amount of visceral fat, gall bladder and spleen enlargement and myocardium dystrophy (Alexakhin et al. 2004).

Changes in the concentration of thyroid hormones and adenylyl cyclase activity in cattle in the first year after the NRE were reversible. This response indicated that there was a compensatory mechanism for the activation of cyclic AMP system in animals with reduced secretion of thyroid hormones in case of thyroid damage (Shevchenko et al. 1990). Concentrations of thyroid hormone were also low during lactation.

The offspring of exposed cows had reduced live weight, but reproductive capacity returned to normal by 1989 (Astasheva et al. 1991). There was no evidence of an increased occurrence of congenital malformations in offspring of cows that were evacuated from the 30 km zone.

The severity of radiation damage to the thyroid was linked with the stable iodine content in the animal's diet. In sheep from the Belarusian Poliessie, a reduced level of iodine nutrition (that commonly occurred in this area) led to the thyroid accumulating a relatively large proportion of the absorbed radioiodine and 2–2.5-fold higher doses to the thyroid than in controls (Budarkov et al. 1992).

Five months after the Chernobyl NRE, many sheep evacuated from the 30 km zone developed serious haematological alterations in the peripheral circulation (Alexakhin et al. 2004). Leucopenia was reported in 89% of animals and lymphopenia in 90%. Also 54% of sheep exhibited initial and marked anaemia and 34% had serious inhibition of haemopoiesis. Offspring of highly exposed cows had reduced weight, decreased daily live weight gains and disruptions to their hormonal status (Astasheva et al. 1991). Reproduction returned to normal in the spring of 1989. No valid data on an increased occurrence of teratogenesis in offspring of the evacuated from the 30 km zone animals was recorded.

Chronic radiation damage was still detected in sheep and horses that had been in a highly contaminated area nearly 2 years after they had been removed. They were generally in poor condition and emaciated and had decreased thyroid hormone levels.

5.8 Routes of Radionuclide Intake via Aquatic Pathways

Radionuclides released after a NRE enter the aquatic environment via a number of routes. When released into the atmosphere, radionuclides will be deposited onto catchments from which there will be an initial transfer through the catchment via runoff, especially if deposition is associated with rainfall, into streams and rivers which will ultimately be discharged into coastal and open ocean marine systems. After the initial period of radionuclide deposition during the emergency response phase, subsequent transfer from catchments occurs through processes such as run-off, erosion, decontamination activities and forestry practices. The rate of loss of radionuclides from catchments may also be enhanced during heavy rainfall events such as typhoons.

After the Chernobyl NRE, long-lived ^{137}Cs and ^{90}Sr formed the major component of contamination of aquatic ecosystems. Fractions of many radionuclides in sediments in aquatic environments may remain in mobile (or exchangeable) states and may transfer from the sediment compartment to the water column (Boyer et al. 2018). The fraction of a particular radionuclide present in these exchangeable phases will depend on numerous factors including, amongst others, the sediment or soil characteristics, the presence of competing ions, pH and redox conditions.

During the first few weeks after the NRE, activity concentrations in river waters rapidly decline, because of the physical decay of short-lived isotopes and as radionuclide deposits gradually became absorbed to soils and bottom sediments. In rivers, due to the constant throughflow of water, there is less contamination in the longer term, since contaminated upper layers of bottom sediments tend to be replaced, particularly in flood conditions.

The reduction in ^{90}Sr and ^{137}Cs activity concentrations occurred at a similar rate for different rivers in the vicinity of Chernobyl and in rivers in Western Europe (Monte 1995). In small catchments, highly organic soils such as saturated peat soils released up to an order of magnitude more radiocaesium to surface waters than occurred where there were mineral soils present (Smith et al. 2004).

In some lakes radiocaesium activity concentrations in water remained relatively high due to continuing inputs of runoff from organic soils in the catchment. In addition, internal cycling of radiocaesium in lakes with little inflow and outflow of water led to much higher activity concentrations in their water and aquatic biota than were typically seen in open lakes and rivers with higher amounts of water inflow and outflow. Radionuclide activity concentrations in water declined rapidly in reservoirs and lakes with significant inflow and outflow of water.

Radionuclides deposited onto lakes or reservoirs are also removed from the water by the sedimentation of particulate material, leading to the long-term removal of radionuclides from the surface layers to bottom sediments. Radiocaesium activity concentrations in lakes decline relatively rapidly during the first months after fallout followed by slower declines over a period of years as radiocaesium became more strongly absorbed to soils and river bed sediments.

In lakes where the radiocaesium originated from organic soil catchments, the contamination was approximately an order of magnitude higher than in nearby lakes with mineral soil catchments (Hilton et al. 1993). Some lakes in Western Europe with organic catchments had radiocaesium activity concentrations in water and fish that were similar to those in some lakes in the more highly contaminated areas in Ukraine and Belarus. Long-term contamination can also be caused by remobilization of radionuclides from bed sediments. In shallow “closed” lakes where there were no significant surface inflow and outflow of water, the bed sediments played a major role in determining radionuclide activity concentration in the water.

5.8.1 Radionuclides in Freshwater Fish

The principal route of accumulation of radionuclides for aquatic animals is via food, but some radionuclides can be directly absorbed from the water. Radionuclide uptake from freshwater is influenced by the ambient chemistry.

Radionuclide activity concentrations in fish vary considerably in different species and depend on physiological features such as mass, dietary preferences and preferred habitat within the water column.

There are only limited data on uptake of ^{131}I in fish. After the Chernobyl NRE, ^{131}I was rapidly absorbed by fish reaching as high as 6000 Bq/kg fw soon after the contamination of water bodies but within approximately 1 month fell to only 50 Bq/kg fw (IAEA 2006a). This represents a rate of decline similar to that of its physical decay. The ^{131}I activity concentrations in fish became insignificant a few months after the NRE.

There have been many studies on radiocaesium contamination of freshwater fish. Because of its chemical similarity to caesium, the potassium concentration of lake or river water influences the rate of accumulation of radiocaesium in fish. Strong inverse relationships were reported between the potassium concentration in water and that of ^{137}Cs in fish (Smith et al. 2002). Bioaccumulation factors in lakes with low potassium concentrations could be one order of magnitude higher than that in lakes with high potassium concentration. Thus, fish from lakes in agricultural areas where runoff of potassium fertilizer is significant had lower bioaccumulation factors than fish from lakes in seminatural areas (Smith et al. 2002).

After the Chernobyl NRE, the accumulation of radiocaesium resulted in activity concentrations in some fish that were above intervention levels for consumption. The elevated levels persisted for many years in some areas in both the most affected regions of the USSR and parts of Western Europe (Jonsson et al. 1999).

There are relatively high transfer and retention of radiocaesium by some fish species, despite low radiocaesium activity concentrations in water. Uptake of radiocaesium in small fish was relatively rapid, with the maximum activity concentrations occurring a few weeks after a NRE (Jonsson et al. 1999; Zibold et al. 2002). Due to the slower uptake rates of radiocaesium in large predatory fish (e.g. pike, eel), maximum activity concentrations took up to a year after the NRE to be established.

In shallow closed lakes, ^{137}Cs activity concentrations in fish declined slowly in comparison with fish in rivers and open lake systems, due to the slow decline in radionuclide activity concentrations noted above. In the long term, ^{137}Cs activity concentrations in predatory fish were significantly higher than non-predatory fish, and large fish tended to have higher activity concentrations than small. The increase in activity concentration in large fish is termed the "size effect" and is due to metabolic and dietary differences. Radiocaesium activity concentration in large predatory fish could be five to ten times higher than in non-predatory fish.

After the Chernobyl NRE, there was a focus on collecting data for radiocaesium from some of the many lakes in Finland. The concentration of ^{137}Cs in pike tissues peaked after only 2 years. Over a 10-year study period, the $T_{1/2}^{eff}$ of strontium was 15 years for pike and perch and 9 years for vendace (Saxen 2004). However, site-specific characteristics of the lakes led to considerable variation in $T_{1/2}^{eff}$ in individual lakes ranging from 7 to 29 years for pike, 11 to 30 years for perch and 7 to 11 years for vendace. Activity concentrations of ^{137}Cs in 20 different species of fish varied considerably even 15 years after initial contamination, ranging from 16 to 6400 Bq/kg (Saxén and Sundell 2006).

In a contaminated, closed lake in Russia, the ^{137}Cs activity concentration was two orders of magnitude higher than in fish in rivers or flow-through lakes in the same region (Travnikova et al. 2004).

Chernobyl fallout ^{90}Sr entered water courses via runoff and remained in the water phase rather than depositing in sediments as rapidly as ^{137}Cs (Outola et al. 2009). Nevertheless, ^{90}Sr activity concentrations in fish in Finland were much lower than those of ^{137}Cs. Stable strontium and ^{90}Sr behave in a similar chemical and biological manner to calcium in freshwater systems. The ^{90}Sr activity concentration in fish depended on the water chemistry with higher accumulation associated with (i) low calcium concentration in the water (i.e. "soft water") and (ii) low electrical conductivity. Radiostrontium accumulated in calcium-containing organs such as the skin, bones, fins and head of the fish (Kaglyan et al. 2008). Depending on the pattern of deposition of radioactive fallout, there were differences in the concentrations in fish from different lakes. In 15 lakes the average ^{90}Sr activity concentration in fish muscle was 20 and 60 times higher, respectively, in vendace (a non-predator species) and perch (mixed habit) than in pike (a predator). After the initial deposition from Chernobyl, it took 3 years for ^{90}Sr activity concentrations to reach a peak in pike. After this, concentrations decreased sharply to pre-Chernobyl levels. In contrast, in non-predatory vendace, ^{90}Sr activity concentrations were highest 1–2 years after contamination (Outola et al. 2009).

5.9 The Risk for Public Health (Placement on the Market for Human Consumption)

5.9.1 Radioiodine

After the onset of the NRE, the most immediate and important potential source of internal exposure to radioactivity is the short-lived radioiodine isotopes such as ^{131}I. Radioactive caesium (^{134}Cs and ^{137}Cs), in contrast to radioactive iodine, has a long half-life (^{134}Cs, 2 years; ^{137}Cs, 30 years).

The role of iodine in human health and the importance of iodine sources have been reviewed by Fuge and Johnson (2015); some of the main points from the review are briefly described here. Iodine is an essential element in the human diet, and a deficiency can lead to a number of health outcomes collectively termed iodine deficiency disorders (IDD). Human intake of iodine is mainly from food with some populations also obtaining appreciable quantities of iodine from drinking water. Plant-derived dietary iodine is generally insufficient alone. Seafood is an important source of iodine, but other inputs are mainly from sources such as the use of iodized salt and dairy produce.

Radioactive iodine (particularly ^{131}I) in food is of immediate concern due to its rapid transfer to milk from contaminated feed and its accumulation in the thyroid gland. I-131 has a relatively short half-life (8 days), so it will naturally decay over a short time frame. If radioactive iodine is breathed in or swallowed, it will concentrate in the thyroid gland and increase the risk of thyroid cancer.

The uptake of radioactive iodine into the thyroid gland can be decreased or prevented by ingestion of stable iodine in the form of potassium iodide pills. Once the thyroid is saturated with iodine, no further iodine can be incorporated. Iodized table salt should not be used as an alternative to potassium iodide pills as it does not contain sufficient iodine to saturate the thyroid. Furthermore, high salt intake may have adverse health effects.

After the Chernobyl NRE, the ^{131}I activity concentrations in milk were particularly high in privately owned dairy cows which were grazing forest clearings and unimproved land in contaminated areas. Initially, information regarding the need to stop the cows grazing such pasture, and to avoid consuming the milk, was less effective for subsistence households. Consequently, people in these households received relatively high radioiodine doses, leading to elevated rates of thyroid cancers in these areas (IAEA 2006a, b). The impact of ^{131}I consumption was enhanced by the deficiency of iodine in the diet of some of the more contaminated areas around the NPP.

5.9.2 Radiocaesium

In contrast to short-lived radioiodine isotopes, radiocaesium (^{134}Cs and ^{137}Cs) has a long half-life (^{134}Cs, 2 years; ^{137}Cs, 30 years).

Over time, radiocaesium can be accumulated in various terrestrial animals, or into rivers, lakes and the sea where fish and other seafood could take up the radionuclides. Animal products from the wild, such as game meat, may continue to be a radiological problem for a long time. Fish and aquatic microflora may bioconcentrate certain radionuclides, but due to the high dilution of radionuclides in water, contamination tends to be confined relatively locally.

Radiocaesium can stay in the environment for many years and could continue to present a long-term problem for food, and food production, and as a threat to human health. If radiocaesium enters the body, it is distributed uniformly throughout the body's soft tissues, resulting in exposure of those tissues. Compared to some other radionuclides, ^{137}Cs remains in the body for a relatively short time.

5.9.3 *Other Radionuclides*

Other radionuclides could be of concern, depending on the nature of the NRE and release of specific isotopes.

References

Akleyev, A. V., Krestinina, L. Y., Degteva, M. O., & Tolstykh, E. I. (2017). Consequences of the radiation accident at the Mayak production association in 1957 (the 'Kyshtym accident'). *Journal of Radiological Protection, 37*, R19–R42.

Alexakhin, R. M., & Korneyev, N. A. (Eds.). (1991). *Agricultural radiology*. Moscow: Ecology. (in Russian).

Alexakhin, R. M., Sarapultsev, I., Spirin, E., & Udalov, D. (1992). Formation of dose burdens to farm animals after the Chernobyl accident and influence of their evacuation on the absorbed doses. *Proceedings of the USSR Academy of Sciences, 323*, 576–579. (in Russian).

Alexakhin, R. M., Buldakov, L., Gubanov, V., Drozhko, Y., Ilyin, L., Kryshev, I., et al. (2004). *Large radiation accidents: Consequences and protective countermeasures*. Moscow: Izdat Publisher. (in Russian).

Arkhipov, N. P., Egorov, A. V., & Klechlovskey, V. M. (1969). Estimation of ^{90}Sr transfer from soil to plant and its accumulation in crop. *Dokladu VASHNIL, 1*, 2–4. (in Russian).

Astasheva, N., Lazarev, N., Khramtsova, L., Drozdenko, V., Chmirev, M., & Zigarenko, V. (1991). *Influence of radiation released during the Chernobyl NPP accident on clinical and physiological status of agricultural animals. Problems of agricultural radiology* (pp. 176–180). Kiev: UIAR. (in Russian).

Beresford, N. A., Barnett, C. L., Mayes, R. W., Lamb, C. S., Howard, B. J., & Wilson, P. (1995). *Radiocaesium variability within sheep flocks in the restricted area of Cumbria. Final report to the Ministry of Agriculture, fisheries and food* (TFS project TO7051jl). Grange-over-Sands: Institute of Terrestrial Ecology.

Beresford, N. A., Barnett, C. L., Crout, N. M. J., & Morris, C. C. (1996). Radiocaesium variability within sheep flocks: Relationships between the ^{137}Cs activity concentrations of individual ewes within a flock and between ewes and their progeny. *The Science of the Total Environment, 177*, 85–96.

Beresford, N. A., et al. (1998). Generic relationship between calcium intake and radiostrontium transfer to the milk of dairy ruminants. *Radiation and Environmental Biophysics, 37*, 129–131.

Beresford, N. A., Mayes, R. W. M., Cooke, A. I., Barnett, C. L., Howard, B. J., Lamb, C. S., & Naylor, G. P. L. (2000). The importance of source-dependent bioavailability in determining the transfer of ingested radionuclides to ruminant-derived food products. *Environmental Science & Technology, 34*, 4455–4462.

Boyer, P., Wells, C., & Howard, B. J. (2018). Extended K_d distributions for freshwater environment. *Journal of Environmental Radioactivity, 192*, 128–142.

Brown, J., & Simmonds, J. R. (1995). *Farmland: A dynamic model for the transfer of radionuclides through terrestrial foodchains (NRPB-R275)*. Chilton: National Radiological Protection Board. 76 pp.

Budarkov, V., Zenkin, A., Arkhipov, N., Junosova, R., Mayakov, E., Amirkhanian, A., et al. (1992). Effects of ^{131}I on sheep dependent on the stable iodine content in the ration, (in Russian). *Radiobiology, 32*, 451–458.

Comar, C. (1966). Transfer of strontium-90 into animal produce. In R. Russell (Ed.), *Radioactivity and human diet* (pp. 247–275). Oxford: Pergamon Press.

Crout, N. M. J., Beresford, N. A., Mayes, R. W., Maceachern, P. J., Barnett, C. L., Lamb, C. S., & Howard, B. J. (2000). A model of radioiodine transfer to goat milk incorporating the influence of stable iodine. *Radiation and Environmental Biophysics, 39*, 59–65.

Fesenko, S. (2019). Review of effects of non-human species in areas affected by the Kyshtym accident. *Journal of Radiological Protection, 39*, R1–R17.

Fesenko, S. V., Colgan, P. A., Lissianski, K. B., Vazquez, C., & Guardans, R. (1997). The dynamics of the transfer of ^{137}Cs to animal fodder in areas of Russia affected by the Chernobyl accident and doses resulting from the consumption of milk and milk products. *Radiation Protection Dosimetry, 69*(4), 289–299.

Fesenko, S. V., Alexakhin, R. M., Geras'kin, S. A., Sanzharova, N. I., Spirin, Y. V., Spiridonov, S. I., et al. (2005). Comparative radiation impact on biota and man in the area affected by the accident at the Chernobyl nuclear power plant. *Journal of Environmental Radioactivity, 80*, 1–25.

Fesenko, S., Isamov, N., Barnett, C. L., Beresford, N. A., Howard, B. J., Sanzharova, N., & Fesenko, E. (2015). Review of Russian language studies on radionuclide behaviour in agricultural animals: Biological half-lives. *Journal of Environmental Radioactivity, 142*, 136–151.

Fesenko, S., Isamova, N., Howard, B. J., Sanzharova, N., & Wells, C. (2018). Review of Russian language studies on radionuclide behaviour in agricultural animals: Transfer to animal tissues. *Journal of Environmental Radioactivity, 192*, 233–249.

Fuge, R., & Johnson, C. C. (2015). Iodine and human health, the role of environmental geochemistry and diet, a review. *Applied Geochemistry, 63*, 282–302.

Garland, J. A., & Wakeford, R. (2007). Atmospheric emissions from the Windscale accident of October 1957. *Atmospheric Environment, 41*, 3904–3920.

Geras'kin, S. A., Fesenko, S. V., & Alexakhin, R. M. (2008). Effects of non-human species irradiation after the Chernobyl NPP accident. *Environment International, 34*, 880–897.

Gulyakin, I. V., & Yudintseva, E. B. (1962). *Radioactive fission products in soils and plants*. M. Gosatomizdat (in Russian).

Heinemann, K., & Vogt, K. J. (1980). Measurements of deposition of iodine onto vegetation and of the biological half-life of iodine on vegetation. *Health Physics, 39*, 463–474.

Hilton, J., Livens, F. R., Spezzano, P., & Leonard, D. R. P. (1993). Retention of radioactive Cs by different soils in the catchment of a small lake. *Science of the Total Environment, 129*, 253–266.

Hird, A. B., Rimmer, D. L., & Livens, F. R. (1995). Total caesium fixing potential of acid organic soils. *Journal of Environmental Radioactivity, 26*, 103–118.

Howard, B. J. (2000). The concept of radioecological sensitivity. *Radiation Protection Dosimetry, 92*, 29–34.

Howard, B. J., Mayes, R. W., Beresford, N. A., & Lamb, C. S. (1989). Transfer of radiocesium from different environmental sources to ewes and suckling lambs. *Health Physics, 57*, 579–586.

Howard, B. J., Beresford, N. A., & Hove, K. (1991). Transfer of radiocesium to ruminants in unimproved natural and semi-natural ecosystems and appropriate countermeasures. *Health Physics, 61*, 715–725.

Howard, B. J., Beresford, N. A., Mayes, R. W., & C.S. (1993). Lamb transfer of ^{131}I to sheep milk from vegetation contaminated by Chernobyl fallout. *Journal of Environmental Radioactivity, 19*, 155–161.

Howard, B. J., Johanson, K. J., Linsley, G. S., Hove, K., Prohl, G., & Horyna, J. (1996a). Transfer of radionuclides by terrestrial food products from semi-natural ecosystems. In *Second report of the VAMP Terrestrial Working Group* (IAEA-Tecdoc-857) (pp. 49–79). Vienna: IAEA.

Howard, B. J., Voigt, G., Segal, M. G., & Ward, G. M. (1996b). A review of countermeasures to reduce radioiodine in milk of dairy animals. *Health Physics, 71*, 661–673.

Howard, B. J., Beresford, N., Mayes, R. W., Hansen, H. S., Crout, N. M. J., & Hove, K. (1997). The use of dietary calcium intake of dairy ruminants to predict the transfer coefficient of radiostrontium to milk. *Radiation and Environmental Biophysics, 36*, 39–43.

Howard, B. J., Strand, P., Assimakopoulos, P., Brechignac, F., Gasco, C., Metivier, H., Moberg, L., Smith, J. T., Tamponnet, C., Trueba, C., Voigt, G., & Wright, S. M. (2002). Estimation of radioecological sensitivity. *Radioprotection – Collogues, 37*, C1167–C1173.

Howard, B. J., Beresford, N. A., Barnett, C. L., & Fesenko, S. (2009a). Radionuclide transfer to animals: Revised recommended transfer coefficient values. *Journal of Environmental Radioactivity, 100*, 263–273.

Howard, B. J., Beresford, N. A., Barnett, C. L., & Fesenko, S. (2009b). Quantifying the transfer of radionuclides to food products from domestic farm animals. *Journal of Environmental Radioactivity, 100*, 767–773.

Howard, B. J., Wells, C., Barnett, C. L., & Sheppard, S. C. (2016a). How knowledge of the gastrointestinal absorption of elements could be used to predict transfer to milk. *Scientific Reports, 6*, 37041. https://doi.org/10.1038/srep37041.

Howard, B. J., Wells, C., & Barnett, C. L. (2016b). Improving the quantity, quality and transparency of data used to derive radionuclide transfer parameters for animal products. 1. Goat milk. *Journal of Environmental Radioactivity, 154*, 34–42.

Howard, B. J., Wells, C., Barnett, C. L., & Howard, D. C. (2017). Improving the quantity, quality and transparency of data used to derive radionuclide transfer parameters for animal products. 2. Cow milk. *Journal of Environmental Radioactivity, 167*, 254–268.

International Atomic Energy Agency. (1994). *Handbook of parameter values for the prediction of radionuclide transfer in temperate environments* (Technical report series N°364). Vienna: IAEA.

International Atomic Energy Agency. (2006a). *Environmental consequences of the Chernobyl accident and their remediation: Twenty years of experience* (Report of the UN Chernobyl Forum Expert Group "Environment". STI/PUB/1239). Vienna: IAEA.

International Atomic Energy Agency. (2006b). *Chernobyl's legacy: Health, environmental and socio-economic impacts and recommendations to the Governments of Belarus, the Russian Federation and Ukraine* (The Chernobyl Forum: 2003–2005 second revised version). Vienna: IAEA.

International Atomic Energy Agency. (2009). *Quantification of radionuclide transfer in terrestrial and freshwater environments for radiological assessments* (TECDOC 1616). Vienna: IAEA.

International Atomic Energy Agency. (2010). *Handbook of parameter values for the prediction of radionuclide transfer in terrestrial and freshwater environment* (Technical reports series no. 472). Vienna: IAEA.

International Atomic Energy Agency. (2015). *Fukushima Report. Radiological Consequences* (Technical Volume 4/5). Vienna: IAEA.

International Commission on Radiological Protection (ICRP). (2006). *Human alimentary tract model for radiological protection*. Annals of the ICRP, Publication 100.

Jonsson, B., Forseth, T., & Ugedal, O. (1999). Chernobyl radioactivity persists in fish. *Nature, 400*, 417.

Kaglyan, O., Gudkov, D., Klenus, V., Shyroka, Z., & Nazarov, O. (2008). Strontium-90 in fish from the lakes of the Chernobyl exclusion zone. In P. Strand, J. Brown, & T. Jølle (Eds.), *Proceedings: Posters – Part 2. International Conference on Radioecology & Environmental Radioactivity 2008 Jun 15–20, Bergen, Norway* (pp. 176–179). Østerås: Norwegian Radiation Protection Authority.

Kato, H., Onda, Y., & Gomi, T. (2012). Interception of the Fukushima reactor accident-derived ^{137}Cs, ^{134}Cs and ^{131}I by coniferous forest canopies. *Geophysical Research Letters, 39*(20), 1.

Kiefer, P., Pröhl, G., Müller, G., Lindner, G., Drissner, J., & Zibold, G. (1996). Factors affecting the transfer of radiocaesium from soil to roe deer in forest ecosystems of southern Germany. *Science of the Total Environment, 192*, 49–61.

Kinnersley, R. P., Goddard, A. J. M., Minski, M. J., & Shaw, G. (1997). Interception of Caesium-contaminated rain by vegetation. *Atmospheric Environment, 31*, 1137–1145.

Kirchner, G. (1994). Transport of iodine and caesium via the grass-cow-milk pathway after the Chernobyl accident. *Health Physics, 66*, 653–665.

Lengemann, F. W. (1970). Metabolism of radioiodide by lactating goats given iodine^{-1} 31 for extended periods. *Journal of Dairy Science, 53*, 165–170.

Lettner, H., Hubmer, A., Bossew, P., Strebl, F., & Steinhäusler, F. (2007). Effective and ecological half-lives of ^{137}Cs in cow's milk in alpine agriculture. *Radiation and Environmental Biophysics, 48*, 47–56.

Lettner, H., Hubmer, A., Bossew, P., & Strebl, F. (2009). ^{137}Cs and ^{90}Sr transfer to milk in Austrian alpine agriculture. *Journal of Environmental Radioactivity, 98*, 69–84.

Menzel, R. G. (1963). Factors influencing the biological availability of radionuclides for plants. *Federation Proceedings. Federation of American Societies for Experimental Biology, 22*, 1398–1401.

Monte, L. (1995). Evaluation of radionuclide transfer functions from drainage basins of freshwater systems. *Journal of Environmental Radioactivity, 26*, 71–82.

Outola, I., Saxén, R. L., & Heinävaara, S. (2009). Transfer of ^{90}Sr into fish in Finnish lakes. *Journal of Environmental Radioactivity, 100*, 657–664.

Saxen, R. (2004). Long-term behaviour of ^{137}Cs in Finnish lakes. In *Book of extended synopses, IAEA-CN-118* (pp. 54–55). Vienna: IAEA.

Saxén, R., & Sundell, J. (2006). ^{137}Cs in freshwater fish in Finland since 1986-A statistical analysis with multivariate linear regression models. *Journal of Environmental Radioactivity, 87*, 62–76.

Shevchenko, A. S., Vakulenko, A. D., & Isamov, N. N. (1990). Increase in activation by prostaglandin E1 of adenilatcyclase in blood cells of animals found in the Chernobyl affected region. *Reports of All-Union Academy of Agricultural Sciences, 11*, 55–58. (in Russian).

Skuterud, L., Pedersen, Ø., Staaland, H., Røed, K. H., Salbu, B., Liken, A., & Hove, K. (2004). Absorption, retention and tissue distribution of radiocaesium in reindeer: Effects of diet and radiocaesium source. *Radiation and Environmental Biophysics, 43*, 293–301.

Smith, J. T., & Beresford, N. A. (2005). *Chernobyl catastrophe and consequences*. Berlin: Springer.

Smith, J. T., Kudelsky, A. V., Ryabov, I. N., Daire, S. E., Boyer, L., Blust, R. J., Fernandez, J. A., Hadderingh, R. H., & Voitsekhovitch, O. V. (2002). Uptake and elimination of radiocaesium in fish and the "size effect". *Journal of Environmental Radioactivity, 62*, 145–164.

Smith, J. T., Wright, S. M., Cross, M. A., Monte, I., Kudelsky, A. V., Saxén, R., Vakulovsky, S. M., & Timms, D. N. (2004). Global analysis of the riverine transport of ^{90}Sr and ^{137}Cs. *Environmental Science and Technology, 38*, 850–857.

Strebl, F., & Tataruch, F. (2007). Time trends (1986–2003) of radiocaesium transfer to roe deer and wild boar in two Austrian forest regions. *Journal of Environmental Radioactivity, 98*, 137–152.

Tagami, K., Howard, B. J., & Uchida, S. (2016). The time-dependent transfer factor of radiocesium from soil to game animals in Japan after the Fukushima Daiichi nuclear accident. *Environmental Science & Technology, 50*, 9424–9431.

Thorell, C. B. (1964). Secretion of radioiodine in milk following a single oral administration in the cow. *Acta Veterinaria Scandinavia, 5*, 217–233.

Tikhomirov, F. A., Shcheglov, A. I., & Sidorov, V. P. (1994). Forests and forestry: Radiation protection measures with special reference to the Chernobyl accident zone. *Science of the Total Environment, 137*(1–3), 289.

Travnikova, I. G., Bazjukin, A. N., Bruk, G. J., Shutov, V. N., Balonov, M. I., Skuterud, L., Mehli, H., & Strand, P. (2004). Lake fish as the main contributor of internal dose to lakeshore residents in the Chernobyl contaminated area. *Journal of Environmental Radioactivity, 77*, 63–75.

United Nations Scientific Committee on the Effects of Atomic Radiation. (2011). *UNSCEAR 2008 report to the General Assembly with scientific annexes*. New York: United Nations.

Vandecasteele, C. M., Van Hees, M., Hardeman, F., Voigt, G. M., & Howard, B. J. (2000). The true absorption of I-131, and its transfer to milk in cows given different stable iodine diets. *Journal of Environmental Radioactivity, 47*, 301–317.

Walters, B. (1988). Chernobyl derived activity in sheep: Variation within a single flock and with time. *Journal of Environmental Radioactivity, 7*(2), 99–106.

Whicker, F. W., & Schultz, V. (1982). *Radioecology: Nuclear energy and the environment* (Vol. 1). Boca Raton: CRC Press, Inc.

Zibold, G., Kaminski, S., Klemt, E., & Smith, J. T. (2002). Time-dependency of the ^{137}Cs activity concentration in freshwater lakes, measurement and prediction. *Radioprotection – Colloques, 37*, 75–80.

6

Risk Analysis and Control in Animal Production Systems

Anne Nisbet

6.1 Introduction

If radionuclides are released into a rural area as a result of a NRE, precautionary advice, including food restrictions, will be issued for places where permitted levels of radioactivity in food may be exceeded. The aim is to minimize the risk of people consuming contaminated food. Within few days, preliminary monitoring data may be available to help inform decisions on whether statutory food restrictions are required. These restrictions identify specific areas where activity concentrations of one or more radionuclides exceed OILs in foodstuffs. The areas subject to food restrictions may be large, and for some long-lived radionuclides, there is potential for a wide range of food production systems to be disrupted for many years, unless some form of intervention is undertaken. The implementation of management options is one form of protective action that will reduce the activity concentrations of radionuclides in foodstuffs to below OILs, thereby providing reassurance to consumers and sustaining production and livelihoods.

6.2 Management Options

Actions intended to reduce or avert radioactive contamination of agricultural products before they reach consumers have previously been referred to as agricultural countermeasures (IAEA 1994). The term 'countermeasure', although widely encountered, is often perceived by stakeholders as being a rather negative action (Nisbet et al. 2005). The term 'management option' has therefore tended to be used

A. Nisbet (✉)
Public Health England, Centre for Radiation, Chemical & Environmental Hazards, Oxon, UK
e-mail: Anne.Nisbet@phe.gov.uk

in recent years to encompass interventions aimed at reducing or averting contamination, or the likelihood of contamination, of food production systems. They are applied across all phases of the emergency timeline.

A large number of management options for use in intensive livestock production, backyard farms and free-ranging animals have been developed since the NRE at the Chernobyl NPP. Some of these options have been adapted and improved for site-specific conditions following the NRE at the Fukushima Daiichi NPP (NEA 2018). To capture relevant information about these management options and record it systematically, a datasheet template was designed (Nisbet et al. 2015). It takes into account criteria that decision-makers might wish to consider when evaluating different management options. A shortened version of the template has been used for the purposes of this book to provide some generic information on the management options that are applicable to animal production systems. This datasheet template can be found in Annex A, Table A1.

Management options can be implemented at different phases following the NRE, from pre-deposition (when there is a threat of release), through the urgent and early phase and into the late phase. Furthermore, the options can be targeted at specific radionuclides or particular contamination pathways, for example, the transfer from pasture to milk and meat, and during the processing of animal products.

Pre-deposition options, as their name suggests, are actions that need to be implemented prior to the deposition. They prevent radionuclides reaching food products by, for example, the closing of air intake systems at food processing plants, the covering of harvested fodder crops and the sheltering of livestock. These options are radionuclide-independent.

Other management options are implemented when the release of radionuclides to the environment has stopped. These options work by either targeting the live animal or one or more animal-derived food products. Options directed at live animals fall into two main categories: those that involve a change in husbandry practice (e.g. provision of uncontaminated feed) and are radionuclide-independent and those that require the use of additives to prevent or reduce the uptake of specific radionuclides into animals (e.g. Prussian blue to reduce gut uptake of radiocaesium). Live monitoring is useful in providing reassurance to consumers that contaminated produce is not entering the food chain. In situations where it is not possible to adequately reduce concentrations of radionuclides in live animals, slaughter (also known as culling) followed by disposal must be considered as a last-resort option. To reduce the quantities of waste, processing of contaminated animal products followed by storage (e.g. salting of meat, and cheese or butter production) can be effective at reducing radionuclides to levels below the OILs.

Many management options are of a technical nature involving some form of physical or chemical intervention to reduce transfer of radionuclides in the food chain. Other management options can be considered to have more societal relevance. These include support for self-help measures by local provision of monitoring equipment and the raising of intervention levels for animal products to maintain traditional farming practices and ways of life.

The placing of statutory restrictions on the marketing of animal products can generate considerable volumes of contaminated biodegradable waste. Appropriate routes of disposal need to be identified, ideally in advance of a NRE. There are many types of disposal routes that can be considered, ranging from relatively simple in situ methods (e.g. landspreading of milk) to offsite commercial treatment facilities (e.g. incineration of animal carcasses).

Table 6.1 provides an alphabetical list of all the management options considered in this chapter. A distinction is made between options directed at live animals and options directed at animal products. There is also an additional category listing options for disposing of waste produce. Datasheets for these management options

Table 6.1 Management options for animal production systems

Category	Subcategory	No.	Management option
Applicable to live animals (15 management options)	Change husbandry practices (10 options)	1	Clean feeding
		2	Live monitoring
		3	Manipulation of slaughter times
		4	Natural attenuation with monitoring
		5	Restrictions on hunting
		6	Select alternative land use
		7	Selective grazing regime
		8	Short-term sheltering of dairy animals
		9	Slaughtering (culling) of livestock
		10	Suppression of lactation before slaughter
	Use of additives (5 options)	11	Addition of AFCF[a] to feed
		12	Addition of calcium to feed
		13	Addition of clay minerals to feed
		14	Administration of AFCF[a] boli to ruminants
		15	Distribution of saltlicks containing AFCF[a]
Applicable to animal products (9 management options)		16	Closure of air intake systems at processing plants
		17	Decontamination of milk
		18	Dilution
		19	Local provision of monitoring equipment
		20	Processing of milk for consumption
		21	Product recall
		22	Raise intervention levels
		23	Restrict entry of food into food chain
		24	Salting of meat
Applicable to waste disposal (9 management options)		25	Biological treatment of milk
		26	Burial of animal carcasses
		27	Burning of animal carcasses
		28	Disposal of milk to sea
		29	Incineration
		30	Landfill
		31	Landspreading
		32	Processing and long-term storage
		33	Rendering

[a]AFCF is also known as Prussian blue

can be found in Annex A, based on published information for the UK (Nisbet et al. 2015) and Europe (Nisbet et al. 2009). The datasheets have been shortened and adapted where relevant to backyard production.

6.3 Radionuclides of Importance

During an NRE a mix of radionuclides will be released. The mix depends on both the type of source and the nature of the NRE. However, generally, ^{134}Cs, ^{137}Cs and ^{131}I are of particular interest because of their likelihood of release and subsequent impact on people. This can be due to external exposure from inhabited surfaces (which is dominated by caesium isotopes) or ingestion of contaminated food products (where exposure is dominated by caesium and iodine isotopes). In food production systems, radioiodine tends to cause severe short-term problems, whilst radiocaesium has a longer-term impact. Both radionuclides had a significant radiological impact following the NPP NREs at Chernobyl and Fukushima Daiichi. There are other types of NREs (e.g. transport accidents and fires at sites holding radioactive materials) that have the potential to release a wider range of radionuclides into the environment. The most important radionuclides considered to pose a threat to food production systems are ^{89}Sr, ^{90}Sr, ^{131}I, ^{134}Cs, ^{137}Cs, ^{238}Pu and ^{241}Am.

6.4 Seasonality and Radioecological Zoning

The seasons of the year when deposition occurs can have a significant influence on contamination levels in animals and animal products and hence the management strategy adopted. This is particularly the case for MS that house livestock for part or all of the year and provide stored feed. This can lead to seasonal variations in radionuclide concentrations in milk and meat (by up to three orders of magnitude) according to the timing of when (or if) animals are fed contaminated feed or return to contaminated pasture with respect to timing of deposition.

6.5 Decision-Aiding Handbooks for Food Production Systems

In advance of a NRE, decision-makers will need to be in a position to construct a strategy for managing contaminated animal production systems. For small-scale, single radionuclide releases, the strategy may comprise one or two management options that could be applied over the first few days or weeks following the NRE. For wide-scale releases of multiple radionuclides, a management strategy is likely to be more complex, comprising a series of management options that could be implemented over different phases of emergency response and affecting several types of production system.

The selection of individual options depends on a wide range of criteria including effectiveness, technical feasibility, impact (e.g. agricultural, environmental and societal) and cost. For any one NRE scenario, only a subset of options will be applicable. However, as each NRE will be different in terms of its radiological composition and impact on the food chain, it is not possible to establish a generic strategy. Consequently, handbooks for food production systems (as well as inhabited areas and drinking water supplies) were developed in close collaboration with stakeholders to aid decision-makers in the selection and combining of management options in the UK (Nisbet et al. 2015) and Europe (Nisbet et al. 2009). The handbooks can be used in emergency response, or as a preparatory tool, under noncrisis conditions, to engage stakeholders and to develop local and regional plans. In addition, the handbooks are useful for training purposes and for application during emergency exercises.

The handbook for food production systems contains an eight-step decision-aiding framework. This comprises various look-up tables aimed at helping those developing the recovery strategy to progressively evaluate the options and eliminate those deemed unsuitable. This informs the decision-making process and provides a short list of options. The datasheets can then be used to provide important supporting information on, for example, effectiveness, feasibility, waste generation and cost.

6.5.1 Decision-Aiding Framework

The eight-step decision-aiding process to support the management of contaminated animal production systems is summarized below.

Step	Action
1	Identify one or more production systems that are likely to be/have been contaminated
2	Refer to selection tables for either milk or meat production systems. These selection tables provide a list of relevant management options, including those for waste disposal
3	Refer to look-up tables showing applicability of management options for each radionuclide
4	Refer to look-up tables showing key constraints for each management option
5	Refer to look-up table showing typical effectiveness of each management option
6	Refer to look-up table showing whether options incur additional doses to those involved in their implementation either directly or through the management of any secondary wastes
7	Refer to individual datasheets for remaining options and note any additional constraints
8	Based on the outputs from Steps 1 to 7, select and combine options that should be considered as part of the recovery strategy

Further guidance on each of the steps is provided in the following subsections.

6.5.2 *Selection Tables (Step 2)*

Color-coded selection tables are presented for milk (Table 6.2) and meat (Table 6.3). These selection tables provide:

- A list of all of the relevant management options for the production system selected, including those for disposal of any waste arisings
- An indication of whether the management options are suitable for implementation in the pre-deposition, urgent, early or late phases
- A color-coded guide to indicate how easy it is likely to be, to implement the management options based on general knowledge of potential technical, logistical, economic or social constraints. The color-coding distinguishes between:

Table 6.2 Selection table of management options for maintaining production of milk

	Pre-deposition	Urgent phase	Early phase	Late phase
Live animals				
Change in husbandry practice				
Clean feeding				
Natural attenuation & monitoring				
Selective grazing				
Select alternative land use				
Short-term sheltering of animals				
Slaughtering (culling) of livestock				
Suppress lactation before slaughter				
Use of additives				
Addition of AFCF to feed				
Addition of calcium to feed				
Addition of clay minerals to feed				
Administer AFCF boli to ruminants				
Distribution of AFCF saltlicks				
Animal products				
Close air intake at processing plants				
Decontamination of milk				
Dilution				
Provision of monitoring equipment				
Processing of milk for consumption				
Product recall				
Raise intervention levels				
Restrict entry to foodchain				
Waste disposal				
Biological treatment of milk				
Disposal to sea				
Incineration				
Landspreading				
Processing & long-term storage				

	Recommended with few constraints.
	Recommended but requires further analysis to overcome some constraints.
	Economic or social constraints; requires full analysis and consultation.
	Technical or logistical constraints; may only be appropriate on a site-specific basis. Requires full analysis and consultation.

Table 6.3 Selection table of management options for maintaining production of meat

Management options	Pre-deposition	Urgent phase	Early phase	Late phase
Live animals				
Change in husbandry practice				
Change hunting season	Red	Red	Green	Green
Clean feeding	Red	Green	Green	Yellow
Live monitoring	Red	Red	Green	Green
Natural attenuation & monitoring	Red	Yellow	Yellow	Pink
Manipulate slaughter times	Red	Yellow	Yellow	Yellow
Select alternative land use	Red	Red	Red	Yellow
Selective grazing	Red	Red	Green	Green
Slaughtering (culling) of livestock	Red	Pink	Pink	Pink
Use of additives				
Addition of AFCF to feed	Red	Red	Green	Green
Addition of calcium to feed	Red	Red	Green	Green
Addition of clay minerals to feed	Red	Red	Yellow	Yellow
Administer AFCF boli to ruminants	Red	Red	Yellow	Yellow
Distribution of AFCF saltlicks	Red	Red	Yellow	Yellow
Animal products				
Close air intake at processing plants	Green	Red	Red	Red
Provision of monitoring equipment	Red	Red	Yellow	Yellow
Product recall	Red	Green	Red	Red
Raise intervention levels	Red	Pink	Pink	Pink
Restrict entry to foodchain	Red	Green	Green	Green
Salting of meat	Red	Red	Pink	Pink
Waste disposal				
Burial of carcasses	Red	Yellow	Yellow	Yellow
Burning of carcasses	Red	Pink	Pink	Pink
Incineration	Red	Yellow	Yellow	Yellow
Landfill	Red	Yellow	Yellow	Yellow
Rendering	Red	Green	Green	Green

Green	Recommended with few constraints.
Yellow	Recommended but requires further analysis to overcome some constraints.
Pink	Economic or social constraints; requires full analysis and consultation.
Red	Technical or logistical constraints; may, or only be appropriate on a site-specific basis. Requires full analysis and consultation.

- Options that would usually be justified or recommended having few if any constraints (green)
- Options that would also be recommended but would require further analysis to overcome potentially serious constraints (yellow)
- Options that would have to undergo a full analysis and consultation with stakeholders before implementation because of serious economic or social constraints (pink)
- Options that would only be justified in specific circumstances following full analysis and consultation due to major technical or logistical constraints (red)

The classification used in the selection tables is intended to be a guide and requires customization at local or regional level by the relevant stakeholders.

So, for milk, the optimum strategy might be as follows:

	Pre-deposition	Urgent phase	Early phase	Late phase
Live animals	Short-term sheltering	Clean feeding[a]	Clean feeding[a] Feed additives Selective grazing	Feed additives Selective grazing
Animal products	n/a	Restrict entry Product recall	Restrict entry	Restrict entry
Waste disposal	n/a	Landspreading	Landspreading	Landspreading

[a]Clean feeding involves the provision of uncontaminated or less contaminated feed

6.5.3 Applicability of Management Options for Different Radionuclides (Step 3)

Most of the information that is available on management options relates to radioactive isotopes of iodine and caesium due to the importance of their radiological impact in previous NREs. For the other radionuclides considered, there are few data to indicate whether a particular management option is applicable or not. Nevertheless, these radionuclides have certain characteristics in terms of their physical half-life, chemical form, mobility in soil and photon energy as well as other characteristics that will give a guide as to whether an option should be considered or eliminated.

Table 6.4 indicates whether a management option is likely to be applicable or not according to radionuclide. An option is considered to be applicable if:

- There is direct evidence that it is effective for a radionuclide (known applicability).
- The mechanism of action is such that it would be highly likely to be effective for a radionuclide, e.g. on the basis of similar chemical, biological or physical characteristics (probably applicable).

The category of 'not applicable' is attributed to an option if:

- There is direct evidence that it is not effective for the radionuclide.
- There is insufficient evidence on the option-radionuclide combination to make a judgement on effectiveness.
- The physical half-life of the radionuclide. Some management options take a long time to organize and implement so may not be appropriate for radionuclides with short half-lives.
- The low environmental mobility or biological uptake of a radionuclide does not justify the degree of disruption that may be caused by some of the more radical options (e.g. select alternative land use, slaughtering of dairy livestock).

Table 6.4 Applicability of management options for different radionuclides

	Radionuclides						
Management options	^{89}Sr	^{90}Sr	^{131}I	^{134}Cs	^{137}Cs	^{238}Pu	^{241}Am
Radionuclide half-life	50.5 d	29.12 y	8.04 d	2.062 y	30.17 y	87.74 y	432.2 y
Live animals							
Change in husbandry practice							
Change hunting season	✓	✓	✓	✓	✓	✓	✓
Clean feeding	✓	✓	✓	✓	✓	✓	✓
Live monitoring	d	d	✓	✓	✓	d	d
Manipulate slaughter time	✓	✓	✓	✓	✓	✓	✓
Natural attenuation (with monitoring)	d	d	✓	✓	✓	d, g	d, g
Select alternative land use	c	✓	c	✓	✓	e, f	e, f
Selective grazing	✓	✓	c	✓	✓	e	e
Short-term sheltering of animals	✓	✓	✓	✓	✓	✓	✓
Slaughtering (culling) of livestock	✓	✓	c	✓	✓	e	e
Suppression of lactation before slaughter	✓	✓	c	✓	✓	e	e
Use of additives							
Addition of AFCF to feed	a	a	a	✓	✓	a	a
Addition of calcium to feed	✓	✓	b	b	b	b	b
Addition of clay minerals to feed	a	a	a	✓	✓	a	a
Administer AFCF boli to ruminants	a	a	a	✓	✓	a	a
Distribution of AFCF saltlicks	a	a	a	✓	✓	a	a
Animal products							
Close air intake at food processing plants	✓	✓	✓	✓	✓	✓	✓
Decontamination of milk	✓	✓	c	✓	✓	a	a
Dilution	✓	✓	✓	✓	✓	✓	✓
Provision of monitoring equipment	d	d	✓	✓	✓	d	✓
Processing of milk for consumption	✓	✓	✓	✓	g	g	g
Product recall	✓	✓	✓	✓	✓	✓	✓
Raise intervention levels	✓	✓	✓	✓	✓	✓	✓
Restrict entry into the food chain	✓	✓	✓	✓	✓	✓	✓
Salting of meat	a	a	a	✓	✓	a	a

Key:
Half-life: d = days, y = years
✓: Selected as target radionuclide (i.e. known or probable applicability)
a: Management option specific for Cs
b: Management option specific for radionuclides in Group II of periodic table
c: Comparatively short physical half-life of radionuclide relative to timescale of implementation of the management option
d: No/low photon energy of radionuclide makes detection difficult
e: Radionuclide has low feed-to-meat or milk transfer, making radical management options inappropriate
f: Low soil-to-plant transfer makes radical management option inappropriate
g: Management option only effective for short-lived radionuclides

Table 6.5 indicates whether a waste disposal option is likely to be applicable or not according to radionuclide. Five criteria were used to assess applicability:

- Volatilization temperature of the radionuclide. This affects options which are carried out at higher than ambient temperature (burning and incineration).
- Mobility of the radionuclide in soil. This relates to options where the waste may come into contact with soil at depth (burial, landfill).
- Physical half-life of the radionuclide. This affects options with relatively long implementation times.
- Uptake of the radionuclide by marine biota (disposal of milk to sea).

Table 6.5 Applicability of waste disposal options for different radionuclides

Management options	Radionuclides						
	^{89}Sr	^{90}Sr	^{131}I	^{134}Cs	^{137}Cs	^{238}Pu	^{241}Am
Radionuclide half-life	50.5 d	29.12 y	8.04 d	2.062 y	30.17 y	87.74 y	432.2 y
Biological treatment (digestion) of milk[#]	✓	✓	✓	✓	✓	✓	✓
Burial of carcasses[†]	a	a	a	✓	✓	✓	✓
Burning of carcasses	✓	✓	d, b	d	d	✓	✓
Disposal of contaminated milk to sea	✓	✓	✓	✓	✓	c	c
Incineration[†] (1100 °C)[‡]	✓	✓	d, b	d	d	✓	✓
Landfill[†]	a	a	a, b	✓	✓	✓	✓
Landspreading of milk and/or slurry[#]	✓	✓	✓	✓	✓	✓	✓
Processing and storage of milk for disposal	✓	✓	✓	✓	✓	✓	✓
Rendering† (150 °C)[¶]	✓	✓	b	✓	✓	✓	✓

Key:
Half-life: d = days, y = years
✓: Selected as target radionuclide (i.e. known or probable applicability)
a: Not recommended due to the potential rapid movement of the radionuclide in the ground after burial, taken to be represented by a soil mobility (K_d) of between 0 and 30
b: Not recommended due to comparatively short physical half-life of radionuclide relative to timescale of implementation of the management option
c: Not recommended due to the potential for the radionuclide to concentrate in marine foods, taken to be represented by a concentration ratio in marine foods (fish, crustaceans and molluscs) of 1000 or more
d: Not recommended as boiling temperature is below temperature of option. Volatilization may occur

[#]: Nuclides placed or deposited onto surface layers of soil – only plant uptake is considered
[†]: Nuclides are considered to be buried under clean soil – only mobility is considered
[‡]: Maximum temperature at which option is carried out. Operating temperature is typically 850–1100 °C and usually 900 °C
[¶]: Maximum temperature at which option is carried out, typically between 100 and 145 °C

6.5.4 *Key Constraints Affecting Management Options (Step 4)*

Management options invariably have some constraints associated with their implementation. To assist in eliminating unsuitable options, major constraints for each option are presented in Table 6.6 taking into account technical feasibility and capacity, timescales for implementation, waste generation and societal needs. If a major constraint is identified, it does not necessarily indicate that the management option should be eliminated but does raise awareness of specific issues that need to be overcome.

Table 6.6 Key constraints for each management option

Management option	Major (key) constraints
Live animals	
Change in husbandry practice	
Change hunting season	Challenges with enforceability and policing
Clean feeding	Availability of suitable housing with water, power supply, straw for bedding and ventilation Availability of alternative clean feed
Live monitoring	Availability of NaI detectors and trained personnel
Manipulate slaughter time	Availability of abattoir or on-farm slaughtering equipment if immediate slaughter is agreed Availability of additional feed and any implications for animal welfare if prolonged slaughter is agreed
Natural attenuation (with monitoring)	It may take a prolonged period of time for the radionuclides to undergo radioactive decay and weathering from land surfaces Availability of monitoring equipment and skilled personnel to take measurements and samples
Select alternative land use	Market for alternative products and know-how
Selective grazing	Availability of less contaminated land in the area
Short-term sheltering of animals	Time between notification and radionuclide release Availability of suitable housing with water supply
Slaughtering (culling) of livestock	Availability of slaughtering equipment and licensed slaughter men Availability of rendering, incineration and landfill facilities for livestock carcasses if large numbers of animals are culled Disruption to and impact on farmers and food industry Resistance from farmers and members of the public
Suppression of lactation before slaughter	None
Use of additives	
Addition of AFCF to feed	Availability of AFCF and identification of feed manufacturing plants that will add AFCF to feed pellets
Addition of calcium to feed	None
Addition of clay minerals to feed	Availability of clay minerals and identification of feed manufacturing plants that will add clay minerals to feed pellets (clay mineral needs to be compliant with animal feed legislation)

(continued)

Table 6.6 (continued)

Management option	Major (key) constraints
Administration of AFCF boli to ruminants	Availability of AFCF and identification of manufacturing plants that will can produce AFCF boli
Distribution of AFCF saltlicks	Not in coastal areas, only where animals are salt-deficient
Animal products	
Close air intake at food processing plants	Time between notification and radionuclide release
Decontamination of milk	Loss of confidence in the food chain May affect nutritional quality of milk
Dilution	May generate mistrust in the food chain and undermine consumer confidence
Provision of monitoring equipment	Availability of NaI detectors and trained personnel; time will be required to manufacture and calibrate monitoring kits and train personnel
Processing or milk for consumption	May generate mistrust in the food chain and undermine consumer confidence
Product recall	Availability of tracking systems to identify potentially contaminated products that may be in the food chain
Raise intervention levels	Loss of confidence in the food chain
Restrict entry into the food chain	Availability of disposal routes for contaminated food products
Salting of meat	May generate mistrust in the food chain and undermine consumer confidence
Waste disposal options	
Biological treatment (digestion) of milk	Capacity of biological treatment facilities for milk which has a very high biological oxygen demand
Burial of carcasses	Availability and suitability of land for engineering a purpose built burial pit Selection of burial site
Burning of carcasses	Availability of suitable sites due to potential for air and water pollution
Disposal of contaminated milk to sea	Identification of long sea outfalls with the capacity to discharge milk, authorization to discharge milk to sea and transportation and offloading at discharge points
Incineration	Availability of commercial facilities able to accept contaminated material and capacity in the area
Landfill	Availability and capacity of commercial facilities for highly biodegradable material
Landspreading of milk and/or slurry	Availability of land for landspreading (not waterlogged, frozen, in nitrate sensitive area) Capacity of slurry tank to store milk at times when land not suitable for spreading
Processing and storage of milk for disposal	Availability of processing plant willing to accept contaminated milk Availability of storage facility
Rendering	Availability of commercial facilities and capacity in the area

6.5.4.1 Technical Feasibility and Capacity

An option is considered to be technically feasible if the equipment, techniques and resources required to implement it are available in the affected area or can be obtained from outside the area in sufficient number. The capacity of or scale on which an option can be implemented is determined by available manpower, work rates for equipment and restrictions in minimum or maximum areas of land or volumes of material that can be treated.

6.5.4.2 Timescales for Implementation

Selection of management options should take into account time-related aspects (e.g. when the NRE happened, the elapsed time, temporal variation in activity concentrations of radionuclides in the environment and their movement through the food chain). In the case of rapidly developing NREs, alerts are only given after the release has started. If the alert comes too late, it will not be possible to implement pre-deposition options such as the sheltering of dairy animals. For some options, the time of year that the NRE takes place can affect applicability, for example, clean feeding is constrained by the availability of stored clean feed, which tends to be lowest at the start of the growing season. Other options such as incorporation of dietary additives into animal feed or boli take time to organize and prepare, so would not necessarily be available in the urgent phase.

6.5.4.3 Waste Generation

It is not just the placing of restrictions on foodstuffs or product recall that creates wastes. Several management options also produce contaminated by-products (e.g. slaughtering of dairy cows, processing of milk and meat), and routes for their disposal must be considered at the point at which the option is selected. The following criteria are important when selecting disposal routes:

- Characteristics of the waste (volume and activity)
- Legislation concerning disposal routes for the waste
- Capacity of disposal facilities
- Impact of disposal on agricultural land and the environment
- Doses to those handling the waste

Disposal routes for contaminated milk include landspreading, anaerobic digestion, discharge through long sea outfalls and incineration. Options for animal carcasses and meat include burial, burning, incineration and landfill.

6.5.4.4 Environmental Impact

Management options can have positive or negative and direct or indirect impacts on the environment. Direct environmental impacts can include changes in biodiversity from changes in grazing pressure brought about by selective grazing and manipulation of slaughtering times. Pollution of watercourses can occur due to inappropriate landspreading of milk. Indirect effects on the environment can happen, for example, when an individual freedom's is reduced by changes to traditional lifestyles, e.g. restrictions on hunting.

6.5.4.5 Cost

It is very difficult to predict the economic cost of implementing management options because of the numerous factors that influence cost. There are direct costs, such as costs linked to lost production, costs from the implementation of options (labour, equipment, consumables, transport, etc.) and costs from the handling of wastes. Indirect costs include those incurred through the impact on the environment and tourism and loss of market share. The magnitude of these direct and indirect costs will depend on many factors such as the time of year of the NRE. NREs occurring at the start of the growing season have larger consequences for food production systems than those occurring after harvest. Also, relevant is the period of time over which a management option is implemented and the scale of the NRE, as costs are proportional to the area of land affected and the type of land use. Costs for remediating intensive agricultural production are likely to be higher than for small-scale production systems.

6.5.5 Effectiveness of Management Options (Step 5)

The primary aim of many of the management options considered for food production systems is to reduce doses from the consumption of contaminated foodstuffs. Options will be chosen if they reduce activity concentrations in milk and meat to below OILs. Effectiveness is influenced by both technical and societal criteria (e.g. application rates, duration of treatments, physical and chemical form of the radionuclide in the environment, biological half-live, timeliness of implementation and compliance in implementation). They will vary therefore according to the prevailing circumstances. Some management options are included as supporting measures (e.g. live monitoring) and do not reduce doses in their own right but provide valuable reassurance.

Experimental work and field-based studies in the regions affected by the NREs such as Chernobyl and Fukushima Daiichi have enabled the effectiveness of various management options to be assessed under field conditions. Effectiveness is generally expressed as percentage reduction in activity concentration in the target medium (food product) following implementation of a management option. Table 6.7 provides a look-up table on the typical effectiveness of management options for a range of radionuclides and animal products. More detailed information on effectiveness is provided in the datasheets (Annex A).

Table 6.7 Effectiveness of management options

Management option	Radionuclides	Effectiveness	Comments
Live animals			
Change in husbandry			
Change hunting season	^{134}Cs, ^{137}Cs	65–85%	Moose and reindeer
Clean feeding	All	Up to 100%	
Live monitoring	^{134}Cs, ^{137}Cs	Up to 100%	Does not remove the radionuclide but can be highly effective at excluding meat above intervention level from food chain
Manipulate slaughter time	^{134}Cs, ^{137}Cs	30–75%	Sheep and reindeer. Highly variable
Natural attenuation (with monitoring)	All	Not applicable	Does not remove the radionuclide. Decay will occur but may take a long time
Select alternative land use	All except ^{131}I	100%	Does not remove contamination but the ingestion pathway is no longer relevant since inedible crops have replaced crops grown for the food chain
Selective grazing	All	50–80%	Milk and meat
Short-term sheltering of animals	All	Up to 100%	Milk and meat
Slaughtering (culling) of livestock	^{89}Sr, ^{90}Sr, ^{134}Cs, ^{137}Cs	Up to 100%	Does not remove the radionuclide but can be highly effective at excluding foodstuffs above the intervention level from food chain
Suppression of lactation before slaughter	^{134}Cs, ^{137}Cs	Up to 100%	Can be considered as 100% effective if lactation is ceased
Use of additives			
Addition of AFCF to feed	^{134}Cs, ^{137}Cs	75–85%	Sheep, goats, cows and pigs
Addition of calcium to feed	^{89}Sr, ^{90}Sr	50%	Milk
Addition of clay minerals to feed	^{134}Cs, ^{137}Cs	50%	Beef

(continued)

Table 6.7 (continued)

Management option	Radionuclides	Effectiveness	Comments
Administration of AFCF boli to ruminants	^{134}Cs, ^{137}Cs	50–80%	Sheep, reindeer, goat and cow
Distribution of AFCF saltlicks	^{134}Cs, ^{137}Cs	50%	Highly variable within a herd or flock. Only effective if animals are salt-deficient
Animal products			
Close air intake at food processing plants	All	Up to 100%	
Decontamination of milk	^{89}Sr, ^{90}Sr, ^{134}Cs, ^{137}Cs	Up to 90%	Electrodialysis Ultrafiltration (Cs only) ~99%
Dilution	All	Not applicable	Does not reduce doses Very effective at reducing volumes of milk requiring disposal
Provision of monitoring equipment	^{134}Cs, ^{137}Cs	Up to 100%	
Processing of milk for consumption	^{89}Sr, ^{90}Sr, ^{134}Cs, ^{137}Cs ^{131}I	50% 80% 100%	Blanching Meat and fish in brine Storage (^{131}I only)
Product recall	All	Up to 100%	
Raise intervention levels	All	Not applicable	Will lead to increase in doses Very effective at reducing volumes of milk requiring disposal
Restrict entry into the food chain	All	Up to 100%	
Salting of meat	^{89}Sr, ^{90}Sr, ^{134}Cs, ^{137}Cs	Up to 80%	Depends on size of pieces of meat, duration of treatment, concentration of salt

6.5.6 Management Options Incurring an Additional Dose to Implementers (Step 6)

Although management options are chosen to reduce doses from ingestion of contaminated produce, additional doses can be received by those responsible for implementing the options, when they are not part of their routine work. These doses are most likely to be received by veterinarians, farmers and those working on the land. Some management options generate secondary wastes that require disposal (e.g. from food restrictions, food processing and the slaughtering of livestock), which may result in workers at waste management facilities receiving additional doses. A number of factors influence the magnitude of the doses received: radionuclides present, exposure pathways and exposure time. In general, the additional doses received from implementation of management options are trivial. Waste disposal options that concentrate and contain radionuclides are those most likely to incur the largest doses and for which a dose assessment should be carried out. Table 6.8 gives a list of management options for milk and meat, showing whether they result in an additional dose to implementers either directly or through the subsequent generation and management of secondary wastes. Table 6.9

Table 6.8 Management options incurring additional doses to implementers

Management option	Incremental dose from management option	Waste produced	Incremental dose from waste management
Live animals			
Change in husbandry			
Change hunting season	✕	✕	✕
Clean feeding	✓	✓	✓
Live monitoring	✓	✕	✕
Manipulate slaughter time	✓	✕	✕
Natural attenuation (with monitoring)	✓	✕	✕
Select alternative land use	✓	✕	✕
Selective grazing	✓	✕	✕
Short-term sheltering of animals	✕	✕	✕
Slaughtering (culling) of livestock	✓	✓	✓
Suppression of lactation before slaughter	✕	✕	✕
Use of additives			
Addition of AFCF to feed	✕	✕	✕
Addition of calcium to feed	✕	✕	✕
Addition of clay minerals to feed	✕	✕	✕
Administration of AFCF boli to ruminants	✕	✕	✕
Distribution of AFCF saltlicks	✕	✕	✕
Animal products			
Close air intake at food processing plants	✕	✕	✕
Decontamination of milk	✓	✓	✓
Dilution	✕	✕	✕
Provision of monitoring equipment	✓	✕	✕
Processing or storage of food products	✓	✓	✓
Product recall	✕	✓	✓
Raise intervention levels	✕	✕	✕
Restrict entry into the food chain	✕	✓	✓
Salting of meat	✓	✓	✓

Table 6.9 Additional doses incurred following implementation of waste disposal options

Management option	Additional dose to implementers	Additional dose to the public	
		Primary waste	Secondary waste
Biological treatment (digestion) of milk	✓	×	✓
Burial of carcasses	✓	×	✓
Burning of carcasses	✓	×	✓
Disposal of contaminated milk to sea	✓	✓	×
Incineration	✓	×	×
Landfill	✓	×	✓
Landspreading of milk and/or slurry	✓	✓	×
Processing and storage of milk products for disposal	✓	×	×
Rendering	✓	×	×

gives a list of waste disposal options, showing whether they result in an additional dose to implementers and members of the public. This information will not necessarily eliminate options but serves to warn the decision-maker that selection of particular options will have implications for wastes and doses, some of which will require further assessment before implementation. It will be important to monitor all locations where disposal of contaminated animal products and carcasses has been carried out.

6.5.7 *Consideration of the Datasheets (Step 7)*

A subset of options remaining in the selection table after Step 6 are those most likely to be incorporated into the overall management strategy. A closer look at the datasheets contained in Annex A will confirm whether any additional constraints might preclude further options from being considered. This can only be done on a site and incident-specific basis, according to the prevailing circumstances and in conjunction with all of the relevant stakeholders.

6.5.8 *Selecting and Combining Options to Develop the Management Strategy (Step 8)*

The management strategy will consist of a number of management options that can be applied either singly or in combination during the pre-deposition phase and/or in the days, weeks, months and even years following the NRE. The strategy is not fixed. It is regularly reviewed and updated according to the effectiveness of the measures, taking into account the views of all the relevant stakeholders. Several hypothetical worked examples have been developed to help illustrate how the decision-aiding framework can be used to select and combine options in the development of a management strategy. These worked examples are presented in Annex B.

References

IAEA. (1994). *Guidelines for agricultural countermeasures following an accidental release of radionuclides* (Technical report series 363). Vienna: IAE Agency.

NEA. (2018). *NEA international workshop on post-accident food safety science – Summary report.*

Nisbet, A. F., Mercer, J. A., Rantavaara, A., Hanninen, R., Vandecasteele, C., Carlé, B., Hardeman, F., Ioannides, K., Papachristodoulou, C., Tzialla, C., Ollagnon, H., Jullien, T., & Pupin, V. (2005). Achievements, difficulties and future challenges for the FARMING network. *Journal of Environmental Radioactivity, 83*, 263–274.

Nisbet, A. F., Jones, A., Turcanu, C., Camps, J., Andersson, K. G., et al. (2009). *Generic handbooks for assisting in the management of contaminated food production systems in Europe following a radiological emergency*. EUR 24457 EN.

Nisbet, A. F., Watson, S. J., & Brown, J. (2015). *UK recovery handbooks for radiation incidents 2015*. Chilton, PHE-CRCE-018. Available at: https://www.gov.uk/government/publications/uk-recovery-handbooks-for-radiation-incidents-2015

7

Information Systems for Animal Production

Joint FAO/IAEA Centre of Nuclear Techniques in Food and Agriculture

Development and dissemination of the information technology throughout the world, as well as the convention potentials for rapid information exchange, primarily via Internet-based platforms, enable for rapid reporting, data collection, data analysis and situation-based decision-making. Such a workflow is especially important in management of rapidly developing emergencies, including NREs. IAEA has already established several such platforms and is intensively working on the improvements and upgrades of the existing ones, as well as on the development of new, sector-specific information platforms. This chapter gives information on the currently existing/developing IAEA platforms for management of NREs.

7.1 The IAEA Unified System for Information Exchange in Incidents and Emergencies (USIE)

The IAEA has emergency contact points worldwide that can use various channels to communicate with the agency through its Incident and Emergency Centre (IEC – https://iec.iaea.org/usie/actual/LandingPage.aspx). The Unified System for Information Exchange in Incidents and Emergencies (USIE) is a secure website maintained by the IAEA to enable countries to exchange urgent notifications and follow-up information during an emergency.

In an emergency, MS require prompt, authoritative and verified information about the situation and its potential consequences. The IAEA's IEC maintains a list of emergency contact points in MS, States Party to the Conventions on Early

Joint FAO/IAEA Centre of Nuclear Techniques in Food and Agriculture (✉)
Animal Production and Health Section, Vienna, Austria
e-mail: i.naletoski@iaea.org

Notification of a Nuclear Accident (IAEA 2002) and on Assistance in the Case of a Nuclear Accident or Radiological Emergency, and in other relevant international organizations. Via the USIE website, as well as by telephone, facsimile, email and video conferencing, the Centre maintains communication with these contact points. The IAEA's Operations Manual for Incident and Emergency Communication (IAEA 2013) outlines the arrangements for emergency communications.

More than 1000 users from over 150 MS are currently registered in USIE. The System not only facilitates the exchange of notifications and information between countries during an emergency; it also allows them to request information or international assistance. USIE is also used by officially nominated INES National Officers, who access it to share information on events rated using the INES (IAEA 2014). While USIE itself is not a public website, information on events obtained from USIE is available publicly on the NEWS website.

To shorten the time needed to share information from national systems to systems used at international level, the IAEA uses the International Radiological Information Exchange data standard (IRIX) as common data standard for information exchange. Developed by the IAEA together with MS and other international organizations, this standard enables the Agency's counterparts to connect their information exchange systems, thereby allowing for an efficient exchange of event details. This is required under the Convention on Early Notification of a Nuclear Accident. Details that can be shared using IRIX include information on the status of nuclear installations, releases of radioactive material and radiation levels measured in the environment. The IRIX standard has also been implemented in the USIE system.

7.2 Decision Support System for Nuclear Emergencies Affecting Food and Agriculture (DSS4NAFA)

Joint FAO/IAEA Centre of Nuclear Techniques in Food and Agriculture International Atomic Energy Agency, Vienna, Austria

In the event of a large-scale accident affecting food and agriculture, the management and visualization of data are crucial for efficient response by food and health authorities. Traditional collection and processing of datasets are presently inadequate for large-scale emergency response due to the analogue style of data transfer (often resulting in human errors for data input) and complex decision-making process (data not presented in an intuitive manner) which in turn prevents swift decision-making. However, advancements in information technology systems have allowed for improved real-time management of large volumes of data and optimized decision-making support.

The Soil and Water Management and Crop Nutrition Laboratory, under the Joint FAO/IAEA Centre of Nuclear Techniques in Food and Agriculture, developed the Decision Support System for Nuclear Emergencies Affecting Food and Agriculture

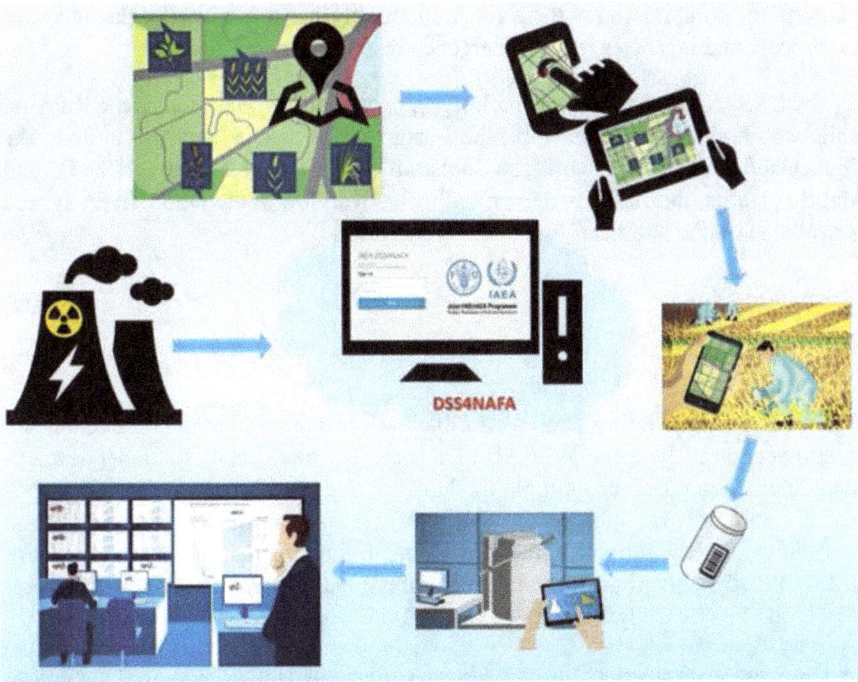

Fig. 7.1 DSS4NAFA is a cloud-based IT tool that assists in data management and data visualization using state-of-the-art technologies

(DSS4NAFA), to assist decision-makers in responding to large-scale emergencies affecting food and agriculture (Fig. 7.1). The specific features that set DSS4NAFA apart is its integrated data management, data visualization and decision support capabilities that assist in overcoming the logistical challenges encountered in a nuclear emergency. The modules in DSS4NAFA supports the logistical assignments of sample collection from the field, sample analysis in the lab, resource optimization and allocation as well as decision support through scenario forecasting. As the system was built such that the data called and time frames set can be customized, the DSS4NAFA system can be used both for nuclear and non-nuclear, routine monitoring and emergency response.

The system platform is accessible on-site through a smartphone application, or via a desktop interface, allowing for streamlined usage and communications. Through the mobile app, which samplers use during the data collection phase, DSS4NAFA allows for reduced human errors and increased information processing speed in the field and lab. Upon obtaining the radionuclide concentration data, the food restriction dashboard collates the information, including the spatial distribution and time resolution of the accident, and suggests food and planting restrictions based on the level of risk and the specified tolerance levels. The use of DSS4NAFA reduces the complexity in managing logistics of data collection, forecasting scenarios in data analysis and proposing restriction actions for decision-making support. The combination of these functionalities brings together all stakeholders in the process and increases robust emergency response capabilities.

The DSS4NAFA system was built using open-source tools such as the Ruby on Rails web application framework, the PostgreSQL/PostGIS database system, the PhoneGap/Cordova framework, the Bootstrap User Interface library and the D3 and MapBox leaflet libraries. A video providing an overview of the DSS4NAFA system is available online at https://youtu.be/Ut4GzjKabMc.

7.3 iVetNet

iVetNet is an online information platform, developed by the Animal Production and Health Section of the Joint FAO/IAEA Division. The platform is still under development and is composed of multiple modules for support of veterinary entities (primarily laboratories) in information management (sharing of standardized operational procedures, SOPs), support in the development, implementation and maintenance of ISO 17025 standard and exchange of professional experiences among the members of the Veterinary Laboratory (VETLAB) network.

The core of iVetNet is the module of competent entities and staff members, attributed with different categorizations, aimed to easily identify institutions/persons competent for management of specific problems of veterinary importance. These include disease diagnosis, management of outbreaks, implementation of disease contingency plans as well as management of emergencies affecting animal production systems, such as the NREs.

The module for exchange of validated SOPs is subdivided into categories, such as procedures for disease detection, vector capturing and identification, procedures for support of ISO 17025 standard (equipment maintenance, staff management, etc.) as well as procedures for response to nuclear emergencies (the management options of this manuscript).

Validated and verified SOPs are shared among the registered users of iVetNet and are permanently available for implementation in their environment. All the procedures, including those aimed for response to NREs, are aimed for integration in the national contingency plans of the veterinary authorities in member states.

Currently iVetNet operates with 112 trial users in 45 member states, most of which (33) are in Africa. The aim of the trial group is to perform "field testing" of iVetNet, identify of gaps and propose improvement measures.

References

IAEA. (2002). *Convention on early notification of a nuclear accident.* https://www.iaea.org/publications/documents/infcircs/convention-early-notification-nuclear-accident

IAEA. (2013). *Operations manual for incident and emergency communication, emergency preparedness and response no. EPR-IEComm 2012.* Vienna: IAEA. https://www.iaea.org/publications/8939/operations-manual-for-incident-and-emergency-communication.

IAEA. (2014). *The use of the international nuclear and radiological event scale (INES) for event communication.* Vienna: IAEA. https://www.iaea.org/publications/10784/the-use-of-the-international-nuclear-and-radiological-event-scale-ines-for-event-communication.

Annexes

Annex A: Datasheets on the Management Options

Anne Nisbet

The list of management options applicable for the animal production systems, as well as their categorisation, is shown in Table 6.1. This annex is presenting the details for each management option, into a standardised datasheet template (Table A1).

Table A1 Datasheet template (Adapted from Nisbet et al. 2015)

Name of management option	
Objective	Primary aim of the option (e.g. reduction of external or internal dose)
Management option description	Short description of how to carry out the management option
Target	Type of object, on or to which the option is to be applied (e.g. soil, crop, animal)
Targeted radionuclides	Radionuclide(s) that the option is aimed at. Radionuclides have been attributed to one of the three categories: **Known applicability**: Radionuclides for which there is evidence that the option will be effective **Probable applicability**: Radionuclides for which there is no direct evidence the option will be effective but for which it could be expected to be so **Not applicable**: Radionuclides for which there is evidence that the option will not be effective. Reasons for this are given
Scale of application	An indication of whether the option can be applied on a small or large scale

(continued)

Table A1 (continued)

Name of management option	
Time of application	Time relative to the NRE when the option is applied
Effectiveness	**Provides information on the effectiveness of the management option and factors affecting effectiveness**
Management option effectiveness	Effectiveness is the reduction in activity concentration in the animal product after applying the management option
Factors influencing effectiveness of procedure	Technical and social factors
Requirements	**Provides information on all of the equipment and facilities required to carry out the management option**
Specific equipment	Primary equipment for carrying out the option
Ancillary equipment	Secondary equipment that may be required to implement the option
Utilities and infrastructure	Utilities and infrastructure which may be required to implement the option
Consumables	Consumables which may be required to implement the option
Skills	Skills which may be required to implement the option
Budget	Indicates whether the cost of implementation is low, medium or high
Waste	**Some management options create waste, the management of which must be carefully considered at the time the option is selected**
Amount and type	Nature and volume of waste (e.g. number of livestock carcasses, volume of milk and amount of soil). Also, indication of whether waste is contaminated and, if so, to what level compared with the original material
Possible transport, treatment and storage routes	Type of vehicle required to transport waste. Requirement to treat waste in situ or at an offsite facility. Options for storage if no direct disposal option Datasheets for waste treatment and disposal options are hyperlinked
Impact	**Provides information on side effects incurred following implementation of the management option**
Environmental	Impact of option on the environment (e.g. biodiversity, pollution)
Agricultural	Impact of option on agricultural practices
Social	Impact of option on behaviours
Practical experience	
Evidence	Widely used. Trialled. Experimental
Key references	
	References to key publications leading to other sources of information

(continued)

Table A1 (continued)

1 Clean feeding	
Objective	To reduce activity concentrations of radionuclides in milk, meat and eggs to below Operational Intervention Levels (OILs)
Management option description	Provide animals with less or uncontaminated feedstuffs. Target animals may be those grazing contaminated pastures or already housed animals which would otherwise be receiving contaminated diets. Clean feeding can be used to prevent animals becoming contaminated in the first place or to minimise the time need for metabolism and excretion to reduce the contamination to an acceptable level Livestock may be fenced in enclosures or housed to prevent grazing of contaminated pasture. The animals are then given nutritionally balanced diets comprising uncontaminated and/or less contaminated feed so that the final animal product has activity concentrations less than the Operational Intervention Levels (OILs). Live monitoring prior to slaughtering provides reassurance to consumers that the clean feeding regime is effective For milk- or egg-producing animals, clean feeding will need to be continuous, while pasture/food activity concentrations would result in milk or eggs exceeding OILs For meat-producing animals, clean feeding is only required for a suitable period prior to slaughter (depending upon initial activity concentrations and biological half-lives). This could be achieved by moving animals onto uncontaminated pasture prior to slaughter, a practice which is already common in some areas (e.g. fattening of hill-bred sheep on lowland pasture prior to slaughter)
Target	All livestock that are destined for the food chain, especially grazing animals
Targeted radionuclides	All radionuclides
Scale of application	Large-scale application, although dependent on supply of suitable clean feed
Time of application	Urgent, early and late phases
Effectiveness	
Management option effectiveness	Will effectively reduce the contamination in meat and milk according to the animal's biological half-life for a given radionuclide. Combination of long biological and physical half-lives will limit the effectiveness of this management option for ^{239}Pu, ^{241}Am and ^{90}Sr if used on contaminated animals A reduction factor of 2–5 (50–80% reduction) is seen for ^{137}Cs and ^{90}Sr from clean feeding (IAEA, 2012)

(continued)

Table A1 (continued)

1 Clean feeding	
Factors influencing effectiveness of procedure	Availability and level of contamination of alternative feeds Rate at which alternative diet is introduced and duration of feeding regime. If grazing stops and the new (less contaminated) diet comprises root crops and cereals, a period of adaptation of 2 weeks is desirable. This is less important if the uncontaminated diet contains silage and hay Biological half-life of specific radionuclide-livestock species combination The requirement for clean feeding and the availability of conserved feed will be dependent on the time of year that a NRE occurs. For example, at the end of the growing season, there would be little impact for housed livestock being fed stored feeds. Finishing lambs grazing forage crops however would have to be housed and given conserved clean feed. Late spring would be the worst time for a contamination event, since cattle and lambs would be grazing outside and no new hay or silage would have been harvested. If the NRE was later in summer, animals could be fed hay or silage that had been cut before the NRE For some of the alternative diets, reduction in grazing is only worth considering for restrictions lasting more than a few weeks because of time required to introduce alternative diets
Requirements	
Specific equipment	Live monitoring equipment Existing farm buildings could be used to house livestock, although some would require modification to penning and feeding arrangements or ventilation. New, purpose-built sheds could also be considered if period of clean feeding warranted this Storage facilities for clean feed. Storage facilities for slurry or manure
Ancillary equipment	Slurry tanks and manure spreading equipment Forage harvester to cut grass for pasture management (see below)
Utilities and infrastructure	Water. Power supply. Ventilation
Consumables	Alternative feeds. Straw for bedding There may be limitations due to the availability of clean feed. For example, with the Fukushima NRE occurring in late spring, there was a problem that the availability of stored feed was limited
Skills	Farmers would possess the necessary skills as looking after housed animals is an existing practice
Budget	Inexpensive if only required for a short period and clean feed is available on the farm Expensive if modification to housing or new housing is required. Also expensive if period of clean feeding is of long duration and supplies have to be brought in from other areas. The time required for farmers to look after livestock not normally housed can be significant The period of clean feeding required will be influenced by initial activity concentration of livestock, biological half-life and activity concentration of replacement feed

(continued)

Table A1 (continued)

1 Clean feeding	
Waste	
Amount and type	A programme of grassland management must be implemented while livestock are fenced or housed to ensure that OILs are not exceeded when the animals are reintroduced to pasture and that pasture quality is maintained. This involves cutting and disposing of contaminated grass before animals are returned to pasture Slurry or manure produced while livestock are fenced in or housed
Possible transport, treatment and storage routes	The cut grass may be composted and the compost subsequently applied to the land Alternatively, silage may be made from the harvested biomass. Such silage could later be fed to noncritical stock or stored for an extended period to allow for radioactive decay. If the critical radionuclide was ^{131}I (or other radionuclides with short physical half-lives), then the normal feed storage period of 6–12 months would more than suffice Slurry or manure should be stored and land spread at appropriate times (i.e. when land is not frozen or waterlogged)
Impact	
Environmental	Housing of livestock produces large volumes of slurry or manure. Inappropriate disposal of this additional slurry or manure could lead to pollution of water courses Possible changes in landscape due to citing of new buildings
Agricultural	Animal welfare issues if animals are housed in the summer when temperature and ventilation could be a problem (e.g. humidity, high levels of ammonia in buildings) Reduced grazing on fields
Social	Disruption to people's image or perception of 'countryside', e.g. if there are no animals in the fields, with potential impacts on tourism, etc.
Practical experience	
Evidence	Clean feeding is still in use in Norway and Sweden due to the Chernobyl NRE for sheep, reindeer and some cattle grazing unimproved pastures Clean feeding was also used following the Fukushima and Kyshtym NREs
Key references	
	IAEA (2012): International Atomic Energy Authority Technical Report Series No 475, Guidelines for Remediation Strategies to Reduce the Radiological Consequences of Environmental Contamination. IAEA, Vienna, 2012

(continued)

Table A1 (continued)

2 Live monitoring	
Objective	To determine whether activity concentration in animals is below Operational Intervention Levels (OILs)
Management option description	Live monitoring can establish the contamination level of gamma-emitters in the animals before slaughtering and can be used to confirm that OILs are not exceeded in livestock destined for the food chain. Live monitoring of animals may be carried out on the farm and also at slaughterhouses. If the activity concentration is above the OIL for animals on the farm, other management options such as clean feeding or addition of AFCF to concentrate ration can then be used to lower the activity concentration before slaughter A rapid, simple, inexpensive and effective method of monitoring contamination for gamma-emitting radionuclides is to use a portable, preferably lead-shielded, NaI detector, linked to (or with integral) single- or multichannel analysers. Adequate shielding of monitors is required to avoid high background counts in highly contaminated areas or areas with high natural background. Equipment needs to be weatherproof (i.e. resistant to low temperatures (potentially to -20 °C) under field conditions); rapid temperature shocks to the detector should be avoided
Target	Meat-producing livestock (e.g. cattle, sheep, goats)
Targeted radionuclides	**Known applicability**: ^{134}Cs, ^{137}Cs **Probable applicability**: ^{131}I **Not applicable**: Radionuclides with no/low effective photon emissions (i.e. beta and alpha emitters, ^{89}Sr, ^{90}Sr, ^{239}Pu and ^{241}Am)
Scale of application	Large scale when monitors are available
Time of application	Early to late phase. A shortage of detectors and trained personnel makes this option more applicable in the medium to long term
Effectiveness	
Management option effectiveness	Can be highly effective (~ 100%) at excluding meat above OILs from food chain
Factors influencing effectiveness of procedure	**Radiocaesium** Accuracy of calibration and detector type. Counting times. Difficulty in keeping animals still during monitoring can lead to erroneous readings Uncertainty on measurements may mean that animals are rejected for the food chain at levels much below the OIL. For example, in the UK a level of 645 Bq ^{137}Cs kg^{-1} in sheep was used instead of the post-Chernobyl intervention level of 1000 Bq kg^{-1}, due to the type and age of the detector used **Other radionuclides** While in theory live monitoring may be possible for all gamma-emitting radionuclides with energy sufficiently high to detect, there is little field experience of trying to determine levels in meat for radionuclides other than Cs **The following may be problematic or need consideration**: Mixed deposits would present problems if using NaI detectors (single-channel analysers)

(continued)

Table A1 (continued)

2 Live monitoring	
Requirements	
Specific equipment	Portable, preferably lead-shielded, NaI detector linked to single- or multichannel analyser with battery supply – calibrated for animals being monitored. Detector and analyser should preferably be as weatherproof as possible
Ancillary equipment	Restraints for livestock (e.g. cattle crush) will be required while monitoring some animals
Utilities and infrastructure	Suitable penned area to contain livestock before monitoring. Good administrative support
Consumables	Paint and ear tags to mark failed animals, or alternative identification method
Skills	Monitoring would be carried out by trained personnel with animal handling experience Ideally, team would consist of two people with farmer providing assistance (catching animals, etc.). More people may be required if large animals (e.g. cattle, horses)
Budget	Expensive (extensive monitoring required) – varies according to scale of restrictions and distances involved
Waste	
Amount and type	None
Impact	
Environmental	None
Agricultural	No direct impact other than a disruption to normal practice A monitoring result in excess of the OIL may result in slaughter or sale times being delayed until activity concentrations fall below the OIL. This represents a loss of flexibility in marketing practice and may also result in the production of overfat animals
Social	None
Practical experience	
Evidence	Combined with clean feeding, live monitoring was the main method of managing the entry of meat into the food chain in the former Soviet Union Used in Norway (from 1987 until 2018) and the UK (from 1986 until 2012) for monitoring sheep from Chernobyl in restricted areas. Soon after the Chernobyl NRE also used for monitoring cattle and goats in Norway Used in Norway (from 1987) and Sweden (from 1988) until present (2014) to monitor reindeer from Chernobyl-restricted areas Used in Ireland and Sweden to monitor carcasses at slaughterhouses, following Chernobyl NRE
Key references	
	IAEA (2012) International Atomic Energy Authority Technical Report Series No 475, Guidelines for Remediation Strategies to Reduce the Radiological Consequences of Environmental Contamination. IAEA, Vienna, 2012

(continued)

Table A1 (continued)

3 Manipulation of slaughter times	
Objective	To reduce activity concentrations of radionuclides in meat (including offal) to below Operational Intervention Levels (OILs)
Management option description	In the early phase, manipulation of slaughter times may be used to minimise the entry of radionuclides into animal products by slaughtering soon after deposition, i.e. before the livestock have eaten so much contaminated feed that meat concentrations exceed OILs. This requires capability to gather free-ranging animals quickly and to transport them to slaughterhouses, and also the capacity to handle more animals at slaughterhouses. Conversely, if slaughtering is delayed to allow for radionuclide concentrations to decline below OILs, the increase in animal numbers on the farm could cause logistical problems with regard to accommodation and also have implications for animal welfare and stocking rate In the longer term, seasonal variation in the radionuclide content of animals diets, and hence meat, may be exploited (i.e. slaughtering occurring at a time of year when the contamination levels are low)
Target	Meat-producing livestock including farmed animals, free-grazing sheep
Targeted radionuclides	**Known applicability**: ^{134}Cs, ^{137}Cs
Scale of application	Small to large scale
Time of application	Early to long term. Urgent, early and late phases
Effectiveness	
Management option effectiveness	Up to 100% if slaughter time brought forward to prevent uptake of radiocaesium to meat If animals graze pastures where fungi are abundant in certain years, the slaughter can be brought forward to avoid mushroom consumption (in some countries). This can give 75–80% reduction in sheep meat contamination when mushroom forms a large part of the diet. Even where fungi consumption is not important, Cs levels in free-ranging sheep are generally higher in summer, so an earlier slaughter time can be effective
Factors influencing effectiveness of procedure	Timing of slaughter compared to deposition Temporal variations in activity concentrations in animal diet Biological half-life, which is animal, organ and radionuclide specific
Requirements	
Specific equipment	Abattoir or slaughtering equipment on farm for immediate slaughter (early phase)
Ancillary equipment	Extra fencing of areas for animal collection and possibly holding until slaughter (in which case water would be required) Live monitoring equipment
Utilities and infrastructure	Transport to take animals to abattoir Storage or deep freeze facilities could be required if large numbers of animals are slaughtered at the same time (especially if used in early phase)
Consumables	Feed for prolonged fattening period
Skills	Slaughtering would be carried out by licensed slaughter men with necessary skills

(continued)

Table A1 (continued)

3 Manipulation of slaughter times	
Budget	Expensive – Costs vary according to scale of implementation Additional cold storage facilities if many animals slaughtered in short time period as early-phase management option Additional feed for prolonged fattening Additional work by abattoir operators or on-farm slaughter men
Waste	
Amount and type	None
Impact	
Environmental	Possible positive impact on biodiversity if grazing period is shortened Possible negative impact if grazing is too intense
Agricultural	**Immediate slaughter:** Lower slaughter weight of young animals if the slaughter is performed earlier than usual. Meat from such animals is likely to have a lower fat content and hence poorer flavour. Furthermore, the conventional jointing of carcasses may not be feasible, and bulk slaughtering of animals is likely to reduce market value. Early slaughter of young livestock may mean that animals that would otherwise have been retained for breeding are not **Planned delay in slaughtering time:** Poorer meat quality if the slaughter is performed later than usual – it will be fatty and tough. There may be a need to change product description, e.g. lamb may have to be classified as mutton. For both younger and older animals, it is likely that a greater than normal proportion of the carcass would have to be used for low-grade meat products, such as mince, sausages and pies, than for prime cuts **Pigs.** Pigs reared and fattened outdoors would be subject to similar constraints as those of ruminant livestock described above. However, the early or late slaughter of pigs may not result in the same penalties with regard to the cash value of the carcass since there are a number of economically viable conventional slaughter weights (i.e. porkers, cutters, baconers and heavy hogs). Thus bringing forward or prolonging the age of slaughter may simply mean changing the slaughter weight category
Social	Altering slaughtering periods can have profound consequences for annual cycles of farming or herding activity, e.g. availability of manpower, provision of feed over longer periods, etc. Disruption or adjustment of farming and related industrial activities, e.g. the supply of meat to food industry and potential market shortages Disruption to people's image or perception of 'countryside' with potential impacts on tourism, etc.
Practical experience	
Evidence	Used in Norway after the Chernobyl NRE for sheep, but other management options like the use of salt licks with AFCF, addition of AFCF to concentrate ration, administration of AFCF boli to ruminants and clean feeding are now dominating Still in use in Norway for reindeer
Key references	
	IAEA (2012) International Atomic Energy Authority Technical Report Series No 475, Guidelines for Remediation Strategies to Reduce the Radiological Consequences of Environmental Contamination. IAEA, Vienna, 2012

(continued)

Table A1 (continued)

4 Natural attenuation with monitoring	
Objective	To allow contamination in animal products to fall below Operational Intervention Levels (OILs) with no active intervention
Management option description	Natural decay of radionuclides will occur with time. When the contamination involves a radionuclide that has short half-life, then simply allowing time for the contamination to decay can be sufficient This option should be carried out in conjunction with monitoring to check on effectiveness
Target	Meat (mainly)
Targeted radionuclides	**Probable applicability:** Short-lived radionuclides such as ^{131}I **Not applicable**: Long-lived radionuclides where no significant reduction in activity level will be seen before a prolonged period of time has passed. Low photon energies of ^{89}Sr and ^{90}Sr may make detection difficult
Scale of application	Any
Time of application	Early–medium term
Effectiveness	
Management option effectiveness	This option does not remove the radionuclide from the affected area; decay will occur, but this may take a prolonged period of time
Factors influencing effectiveness of procedure	Properties of radionuclide; soil type and rainfall (weathering)
Requirements	
Specific equipment	Monitoring equipment
Ancillary equipment	None
Utilities and infrastructure	None
Consumables	Any consumables required for sampling, monitoring and analysis work
Skills	Skilled personnel to carry out sampling, monitoring, analysis and data interpretation
Budget	Expensive (requires extensive monitoring)
Waste	
Amount and type	None
Impact	
Environmental	None
Agricultural	May result in agricultural land being unusable for a prolonged period of time
Social	Potential for public mistrust in authorities over decision to 'do nothing', although monitoring may improve consumer confidence
Practical experience	
Evidence	Large volumes of milk required disposal after the Windscale fire (1957) as the authorities relied on natural attenuation of ^{131}I to reduce activity concentrations in milk

(continued)

Table A1 (continued)

4 Natural attenuation with monitoring	
Key references	
	H. J. Dunster, H. Howells and W. L. Templeton (2007). District Surveys following the Windscale Incident, October 1957. J. Radiol. Prot. 27 (2007) 217–230 IAEA (2014) The follow-up IAEA International Mission on Remediation of Large Contaminated Areas Off-Site the Fukushima Daiichi Nuclear Power Plant. Tokyo and Fukushima Prefecture, Japan. 14–21 October 2013. Final report 23/01/2014

5 Restrictions on hunting	
Objective	To reduce consumption of contaminated meat by restricting hunting to certain times of the year when activity concentrations of radionuclides are low
Management option description	Due to seasonal variation in the diet, the contamination levels in some game species will vary significantly with season. In particular, radiocaesium activity concentrations in muscle of game from areas where fungi can be abundant in certain years can be much higher than the average annual values. By changing or restricting the hunting season to the time of year when contamination levels in the game meat are not enhanced due to dietary preferences, the ingestion dose to humans consuming game meat will be reduced. A short-term ban or a delay in hunting may be applicable to avoid impact of surface deposition of radionuclides on to plants and to allow decay of short-lived radionuclides. This option should be carried out in conjunction with monitoring to check on effectiveness
Target	Those involved in hunting game for the food chain
Targeted radionuclides	**Known applicability**: ^{134}Cs, ^{137}Cs
Scale of application	Large
Time of application	Early to long term
Effectiveness	
Management option effectiveness	Varying hunting times can achieve a 50–70% reduction in radiocaesium activity concentrations in moose meat, with even higher reductions (up to 80%) for meat from roe deer, wild boar
Factors influencing effectiveness of procedure	Successful communication of information regarding the restrictions (e.g. through associations or societies). Compliance with the restrictions. Measurement or prior knowledge to predict times when contamination levels in meat would be lowest (based on contamination levels in diet of game animals)
Requirements	
Specific equipment	Monitoring equipment
Ancillary equipment	None
Utilities and infrastructure	Communication to inform those about restrictions and 'policing' to ensure compliance
Consumables	Dependent on communication method, e.g. leaflets

(continued)

Table A1 (continued)

5 Restrictions on hunting	
Skills	Monitoring. Communication
Budget	Expensive (requires extensive monitoring)
Waste	
Amount and type	If a management programme is initiated that involves culling to maintain stocks at appropriate levels, then contaminated carcasses would require disposal
Possible transport, treatment and storage routes	Slaughtering (culling) of livestock followed by rendering, burning, burial or incineration
Impact	
Environmental	Impact on the ecosystem, population dynamics, breeding, etc. The number of game animals must be kept at a sustainable level. It is therefore important to cull animals even if the meat does not enter the food chain
Agricultural	Possible increase in grazing of agricultural land if hunting season is delayed and alternative food sources are scarce. If hunting is carried out earlier than normal, lower slaughter weights may be expected
Social	Loss of traditional activities. Possible negative psychological impact necessitating good communication programme
Practical experience	
Evidence	A change of hunting season was used in the former USSR and some Nordic countries (such as Norway and Sweden) following the Chernobyl NRE
Key references	
	IAEA (2012) International Atomic Energy Authority Technical Report Series No 475, Guidelines for Remediation Strategies to Reduce the Radiological Consequences of Environmental Contamination. IAEA, Vienna, 2012

6 Select alternative land use	
Objective	To allow agricultural land to be used for productive activities by selecting crops or animals for the production of non-edible products
Management option description	Contaminated land may be used for non-food production, such as flax for fibre; rapeseed for bio-diesel; sugar beet for bioethanol; and perennial grasses or coppice for biofuel. Agricultural land may also be used for the production of leather and wool. In extreme situations land may be used for forestry or given over to recreational use (e.g. golf courses). There must be a market for alternative products or enterprises. Monitoring of non-food products will be required for reassurance of the public
Target	Land used for livestock (milk, meat and egg production)
Targeted radionuclides	**Known applicability**: ^{134}Cs, ^{137}Cs **Probable applicability**: ^{90}Sr **Not applicable**: Short physical half-lives of ^{89}Sr and ^{131}I may preclude this radical option

(continued)

Table A1 (continued)

6 Select alternative land use	
Scale of application	Large
Time of application	Long-term
Effectiveness	
Management option effectiveness	This option does not remove contamination, but as the ingestion pathway is no longer relevant, it can be considered 100% effective
Factors influencing effectiveness of procedure	Expertise in growing alternative crops and supporting different livestock. Ease of substitution of non-edible crops for farmer and associated industries
Requirements	
Specific equipment	Sowing or harvesting equipment for alternative land use
Ancillary equipment	None
Utilities and infrastructure	Processing facilities for alternative products
Consumables	Depends on alternative enterprise chosen
Skills	Expertise in cultivation of alternative crop or livestock
Budget	Expensive (new equipment, livestock), according to new land use selected
Waste	
Amount and type	Depends on alternative land use. There could still be contaminated by-products from, e.g. the refining of rapeseed and sugar beet. In the case of change to leather production, meat will need to be disposed of
Possible transport, treatment and storage routes	On-site treatment plants, incineration and landfill
Impact	
Environmental	Change in ecosystem
Agricultural	Change in crop or animal type. Changes in land management and nutrient status
Social	Disruption or adjustment of farming and related industrial activities or maintenance of farming and associated communities. Alternative practices may not be as economically viable (e.g. wool and leather production versus normal animal production regimes). Maintains some income to the farmer. In communities affected by overproduction, diversification may be advantageous
Practical experience	
Evidence	Existing commercial processes
Key references	

(continued)

Table A1 (continued)

7 Selective grazing regime	
Objective	To reduce activity concentrations of radionuclides in meat, milk and eggs to below Operational Intervention Levels (OILs)
Management option description	Optimising the grazing management of farm animals so that pastures with the least contaminated vegetation are used in the most appropriate way. For instance, for dairy (rather than meat animals) or for meat animals before slaughter to allow contamination levels to fall to below OILs at slaughter Animals can also be moved from highly contaminated farms to pastures on farms with lower activity concentrations in vegetation. Livestock can be physically excluded from highly contaminated areas by erection of temporary fences
Target	Meat-, milk- and egg-producing animals
Targeted radionuclides	**Known applicability**: ^{134}Cs, ^{137}Cs **Probable applicability**: ^{89}Sr, ^{90}Sr **Not applicable**: The relatively short physical half-lives of ^{131}I may preclude this time-consuming management option. Low feed to meat transfer of the following radionuclides makes implementation of this management option unnecessary: ^{239}Pu, ^{241}Am
Scale of application	Large
Time of application	Medium–long term (it takes time to organise, which precludes implementation in early phase)
Effectiveness	
Management option effectiveness	Can be highly effective (up to 100%)
Factors influencing effectiveness of procedure	Initial activity concentration in animals, biological half-life of radionuclide and activity concentrations in vegetation on the pasture animals are removed The availability of land providing less contaminated pasture – the area of cultivated grasslands is limited and usually commensurate with the normal stocking rate of livestock for each farm
Requirements	
Specific equipment	Monitoring equipment to assess contamination status of land
Ancillary equipment	Fences. Transportation of livestock to less contaminated areas
Utilities and infrastructure	None
Consumables	Fuel for transportation and construction machinery
Skills	Farmer should have necessary skills
Budget	Inexpensive if livestock are transferred to less contaminated areas on the same farm Becomes more expensive if fencing has to be erected to prevent animals grazing contaminated pasture. Costs also rise if animals have to be transported to less contaminated farms outside the affected area
Waste	
Amount and type	None
Impact	
Environmental	Change in biodiversity of fenced area
Agricultural	Under-grazing of fenced areas of pasture

(continued)

Table A1 (continued)

7 Selective grazing regime	
Social	Disruption to farming and other related activities (e.g. tourism)
Practical experience	
Evidence	Used widely in the former Soviet Union and Norway. Used in the uplands of UK, in combination with live monitoring, to prove that activity concentrations in lamb < OIL
Key references	
	IAEA (2012) International Atomic Energy Authority Technical Report Series No 475, Guidelines for Remediation Strategies to Reduce the Radiological Consequences of Environmental Contamination. IAEA, Vienna, 2012

8 Short-term sheltering of animals	
Objective	To avoid or limit contamination of food products derived from outdoor animals by reducing the ingestion of contaminated feed during and soon after the passage of the plume
Management option description	Short-term housing of grazing animals prior to deposition and feeding with stored feedstuffs. This management option targets dairy animals to reduce the volumes of contaminated milk (and subsequently waste milk requiring treatment). Contaminated meat is not such a short-term issue – clean feeding and changing slaughter time are likely to be more appropriate
Target	All outdoor milk-, meat- or egg-producing animals
Targeted radionuclides	All radionuclides
Scale of application	Potentially large scale depending on farming practices
Time of application	Pre-deposition phase, as soon as the risk becomes apparent
Effectiveness	
Management option effectiveness	Up to 100%
Factors influencing effectiveness of procedure	Time between notification and deposition may limit the feasibility of this option Availability of housing and conserved feedstuffs at certain times of the year Type of housing will determine exposure to airborne radionuclides (e.g. some housing, especially in Southern European countries, is likely to be of a more open construction, and therefore inhalation of radionuclides will still occur) Reluctance of farmers to be outside while there is a risk of contamination which is made if the measure coincides with advice for public sheltering or evacuation
Requirements	
Specific equipment	N/A
Ancillary equipment	N/A
Utilities and infrastructure	Suitable housing with water supply and power if required
Consumables	Stored feed. Bedding (straw, etc.)

(continued)

Table A1 (continued)

8 Short-term sheltering of animals	
Skills	Farmers would possess the necessary skills as housing animals is general practice
Budget	Inexpensive (stored feed, bedding, extra time for farmer)
Waste	
Amount and type	Manure and/or slurry
Possible transport, treatment and storage routes	Normal routes as only small quantities
Impact	
Environmental	None
Agricultural	Rapid change of diet from pasture to stored feed may lead to reduced productivity Animal welfare issues associated with housing animals at unusual times (e.g. temperature and ventilation)
Social	None
Practical experience	
Evidence	Potential efficiency demonstrated in those countries where animals were still housed at time of Chernobyl NRE (e.g. Norway, Finland)
Key references	

9 Slaughtering (culling) of livestock	
Objective	To remove the source of contaminated milk/meat from the food chain
Management option description	Slaughtering could be considered for those animals whose milk/meat would, because of unavailability of clean feed (or other appropriate management option), be so contaminated that it would be considered unfit for human consumption for a significant proportion of their productive life It could also be considered on animal welfare grounds in areas where stockkeepers were evacuated leaving animals un-milked and possibly unfed It is possible that following a large-scale NRE, killing by free bullet (i.e. by a marksman in the field using rifle, shotgun or humane killer) or chemical euthanasia would be the primary method of culling considered initially (on farm or abattoir). Other options would include culling an animal on the farm or at a knacker's yard using a bullet and gun Condemnation completely removes contaminated food from the market but can leave large quantities of animal waste needing disposal
Target	Dairy-, egg- or meat-producing animals
Targeted radionuclides	**Known applicability**: ^{89}Sr, ^{90}Sr, ^{134}Cs, ^{137}Cs **Not applicable**: The relatively short physical half-life of ^{131}I, and/or low transfers of ^{239}Pu and ^{241}Am from feed to milk/meat, is likely to preclude use of this radical option
Scale of application	Small to medium scale depending on severity of NRE
Time of application	Early to medium term

(continued)

Table A1 (continued)

9 Slaughtering (culling) of livestock	
Effectiveness	
Management option effectiveness	Highly effective (i.e. 100%) at removing contaminated meat from the food chain
Factors influencing effectiveness of procedure	Acceptability of and compliance with management option Availability of licensed slaughter men to visit farms in immediate aftermath of NRE Availability of transport to take dairy animals to abattoirs In wide-scale incidents movement of animals may risk the spread of contamination
Requirements	
Specific equipment	Abattoir or slaughtering equipment on farm
Ancillary equipment	Vehicles for transport of livestock to abattoir if necessary
Utilities and infrastructure	Disposal routes for carcasses, e.g. incinerators, rendering plants, burning/burial sites Good routes of communication including opportunities for dialogue with affected farmers
Consumables	Fuel for transport to abattoir if necessary Cartridges for captive bolts, etc.
Skills	Slaughtering would be carried out by licensed slaughter men with necessary skills
Budget	Cost varies according to numbers of animals being slaughtered and subsequent disposal route selected. Compensation costs also depend on scale
Waste	
Amount and type	Condemned livestock carcasses Animal bodily fluids and faeces will need to be managed at the place of slaughter
Possible transport, treatment and storage routes	Disposal by rendering, incineration, burial and burning
Impact	
Environmental	Indirect effect depends on disposal route selected for carcasses. Potential for contamination of surface waters due to run-off from carcasses
Agricultural	If the entire herd or flock is slaughtered, under-grazing of pasture will occur
Social	Negative psychological impact especially on farming community Market shortages if carried out on a large scale Stigma associated with the area affected Disruption of farming and associated industries, impact on people's image of 'countryside', e.g. if there are no animals in the fields, with potential impacts on tourism

(continued)

Table A1 (continued)

9 Slaughtering (culling) of livestock	
Practical experience	
Evidence	Slaughtering of cattle has been carried out in the UK and other European countries following the condemnation of beef because of BSE On a larger scale, there has been slaughter and burning or burial of complete farm stocks (ruminants and pigs) as a consequence of the foot and mouth epidemic in the UK. Herds and flocks were also slaughtered and disposed of in many other MS, including France, Belgium, Germany and the Netherlands Cattle (95,500) and pigs (23,000) were slaughtered between May and July 1986, following the Chernobyl NRE. Many carcasses were buried, and some were stored in refrigerators, but this produced great hygiene, practical and economic difficulties (IAEA, 2006)
Key references	
	Smith J, Nisbet AF, Mercer JA, Brown J and Wilkins BT (2002). Management options for food production systems affected by a nuclear accident: Options for minimising the production of contaminated milk. Chilton, NRPB-W8 International Atomic Energy Authority (2006) Environmental Consequence of the Chernobyl NRE and Their Remediation: Twenty Years of Experience. Report of the Chernobyl Forum Expert Group 'Environment'. International Atomic Energy Authority, Vienna

10 Suppression of lactation before slaughter	
Objective	To reduce the volume of milk requiring disposal before dairy animals are slaughtered
Management option description	If a decision has been made to slaughter dairy livestock because the period of lost production is too long, methods for suppressing lactation should be used to reduce volumes of waste milk requiring disposal. Synthetic oestrogens are effective at inhibiting milk production, although many forms are currently banned by the EU for food--producing animals unless a decision has been made to slaughter the animals. Progestogens or prostaglandins could also be considered The more natural method of drying off involves the abrupt cessation of milking, accompanied by provision of poor-quality feed, removal of concentrates from the diet and restricted access to water. For high--yielding cows the drying off method would be to reduce the frequency of milking over a 2-week period
Target	Dairy animals
Targeted radionuclides	**Known applicability**: ^{89}Sr, ^{90}Sr, ^{134}Cs, ^{137}Cs **Not applicable**: The relatively short physical half-lives and/or low transfers from feed to milk are likely to preclude use of this radical management option for ^{131}I, ^{239}Pu and ^{241}Am
Scale of application	Small to large
Time of application	Early to medium term

(continued)

Table A1 (continued)

10 Suppression of lactation before slaughter	
Effectiveness	
Management option effectiveness	Both hormone treatments and drying off naturally can be considered as 100% effective if lactation is ceased. The time taken to achieve this depends on the method adopted but can take up to 2 weeks. The shorter the period that drying off is achieved over, the greater the potential for animal welfare problems to evolve Suppression of lactation can also be regarded as being highly effective if the rate of milk production is greatly reduced but not ceased
Factors influencing effectiveness of procedure	The method used to suppress lactation. If hormonal, the type of treatment selected The daily milk yield or stage of lactation of the dairy animal
Requirements	
Specific equipment	None
Ancillary equipment	None
Utilities and infrastructure	None
Consumables	Synthetic oestrogens, progestogens or prostaglandins Long-acting antibiotic for udders (in case of mastitis) if more natural methods of drying off used
Skills	Farmers would possess necessary skills for drying off 'naturally' in preparation for calving, lambing or kidding. Some instruction may be required for administering hormonal treatments
Budget	Inexpensive (just requires synthetic oestrogens, progestogens or prostaglandins). Farmer would be paid compensation for subsequent slaughter of each animal
Waste	
Amount and type	Milk contaminated with radionuclides will be produced until milk production ceases. Levels are likely to be in excess of the OIL and will require disposal. If synthetic oestrogens have been used, all milk will require disposal irrespective of radionuclide content
Possible transport, treatment and storage routes	Disposal by landspreading, biological treatment, processing into a milk product suitable for storage prior to disposal and disposal to sea
Impact	
Environmental	Impact only if waste milk is allowed to contaminate waterways as synthetic oestrogens are known to persist causing endocrine disruption to fish
Agricultural	Animal welfare issues. Therefore, immediate slaughter would be preferable Loss of milk production
Social	Disruption of milk supply to the food industry and possible market shortages Negative psychological impact on farmers
Practical experience	
Evidence	None

(continued)

Table A1 (continued)

10 Suppression of lactation before slaughter	
Key references	
	Smith J, Nisbet AF, Mercer JA, Brown J and Wilkins BT (2002). Management options for food production systems affected by a nuclear accident: Options for minimising the production of contaminated milk. Chilton, NRPB-W8

11 Addition of AFCF to feed	
Objective	To reduce activity concentrations of radiocaesium in meat, milk and eggs to below Operational Intervention Levels (OILs)
Management option description	Ammonium-ferric-hexacyano-ferrate (AFCF, Giese-salt, Prussian blue) is an effective radiocaesium binder, which may be added to the diet of dairy cows, sheep and goats as well as meat- or egg-producing animals to reduce radiocaesium transfer to milk and meat by reducing absorption in the gut. It can be added to the diet of animals as a powder or incorporated into pelleted feed. Dairy animals are generally fed a concentrate ration when they are milked (usually twice daily) – incorporation of AFCF into the concentrate ration would allow administration daily. Meat-producing animals would only need to be fed AFCF concentrates for a suitable period prior to slaughter. Live monitoring prior to slaughtering provides reassurance to consumers that this is an effective option
Target	Meat-, milk- and egg-producing animals
Targeted radionuclides	**Known applicability:** ^{134}Cs, ^{137}Cs
Scale of application	Large
Time of application	Medium to long term (requirement to obtain and distribute AFCF makes it unlikely to be applicable to early phase)
Effectiveness	
Management option effectiveness	

Livestock	**AFCF application rate (g/d)**	**Effectiveness (%)**
Sheep	1 g/d	Up to 87%
Goats	1.5 g/d	Up to 75%
Cows: Milk/meat	3 g/d	Up to 83%
Pigs	1.5–2.0 g/d	Up to 85%

Factors influencing effectiveness of procedure	Initial activity concentration and the biological half-life of radiocaesium in the animal Greater effectiveness when farmer or herders use commercially prepared concentrates. Effectiveness may be more variable if mixed as a powder into home-produced rations
Requirements	
Specific equipment	None
Ancillary equipment	None
Utilities and infrastructure	Concentrate manufacturing plants with the ability to add AFCF to feed pellets. Current production facilities for AFCF may be rate limiting if large quantities required
Consumables	Concentrates with AFCF

(continued)

Table A1 (continued)

11 Addition of AFCF to feed	
Skills	Farmers or herders would possess the necessary skills
Budget	Expensive as new manufacturing process and distribution system are required
Waste	
Amount and type	None
Impact	
Environmental	None
Agricultural	Change in production status for organic farms
Social	May increase consumer confidence through effective management
Practical experience	
Evidence	Used frequently after the Chernobyl NRE in Norway for cows, goats and reindeer; in the former Soviet Union, a different compound (ferrocyn) has been used
Key references	
	IAEA (2012) International Atomic Energy Authority Technical Report Series No 475, Guidelines for Remediation Strategies to Reduce the Radiological Consequences of Environmental Contamination. IAEA, Vienna, 2012

12 Addition of calcium to feed	
Objective	To reduce the activity concentration of radiostrontium in milk and other animal produce below Operational Intervention Levels (OILs)
Management option description	The absorption of radiostrontium from an animal's diet is controlled by the level of dietary calcium intake. In the short-term Ca, intakes could be enhanced by farmers adding Ca supplement to feed directly which is given at milking time. In the longer term, it may be more efficient and effective to incorporate enhanced Ca into pelleted feeds during manufacture. Live monitoring prior to slaughtering provides reassurance to consumers that the clay minerals are an effective option
Target	Primarily aimed at milk-producing animals but may also benefit animals used for meat or egg production. Cannot be fed on a daily basis to free-grazing animals
Targeted radionuclides	**Known applicability**: ^{89}Sr, ^{90}Sr
Scale of application	Large
Time of application	Medium to long term (requirement to manufacture and distribute Ca-enriched feeds makes it unlikely to be applicable to early phase)
Effectiveness	
Management option effectiveness	Doubling of calcium intake results in reductions of approximately 50% in the transfer of radiostrontium to milk
Factors influencing effectiveness of procedure	Animal's calcium requirements and prior intake of calcium. High levels of calcium intake can influence the absorption of other essential nutrients; the dietary Ca/P ratio should not exceed 7:1 for prolonged periods

(continued)

Table A1 (continued)

12 Addition of calcium to feed	
Requirements	
Specific equipment	None
Ancillary equipment	None
Utilities and infrastructure	Most likely to be fed with concentrate during milking
Consumables	Calcium supplements or pelleted concentrates with enriched levels of calcium
Skills	Farmers would already possess the necessary skills because of experience with other additives
Budget	Expensive if incorporated into pelleted feed. Less expensive if famers add calcium to feed on the farm
Waste	
Amount and type	None
Impact	
Environmental	None
Agricultural	Change in production status for organic farms
Social	May increase consumer confidence through effective management
Practical experience	
Evidence	Was used following the Kyshtym NRE in 1957
Key references	
	IAEA (2012) International Atomic Energy Authority Technical Report Series No 475, Guidelines for Remediation Strategies to Reduce the Radiological Consequences of Environmental Contamination. IAEA, Vienna, 2012

13 Addition of clay minerals to feed	
Objective	To reduce activity concentrations of radiocaesium in meat, milk or eggs to below Operational Intervention Levels (OILs)
Management option description	Clay minerals (i.e. bentonites, vermiculites, zeolites) can be added to fodder to reduce gut uptake of radiocaesium by farmed livestock. Live monitoring prior to slaughtering provides reassurance to consumers that the clay minerals are an effective option
Target	Meat- and milk- or egg-producing animals. Cannot be fed routinely to free-grazing animals
Targeted radionuclides	**Known applicability:** ^{134,}Cs, ^{137}Cs
Scale of application	Large
Time of application	Medium to long term (securing suitable sources of clay minerals and incorporation into pelleted rations means this option is unlikely to be feasible in the short term)

(continued)

Table A1 (continued)

13 Addition of clay minerals to feed	
Effectiveness	
Management option effectiveness	Bentonite is moderately effective at reducing levels of radiocaesium in milk and meat of various animals. For radiocaesium, reductions of ~50% can be achieved by a dose of about 0.5 g kg^{-1} body weight per day. A maximum reduction of about fivefold can be achieved by a dose of about 1–2 g kg^{-1} body weight per day. However, loss of appetite and weight has been observed if too much clay is given
Factors influencing effectiveness of procedure	Initial activity concentration and the biological half-life of radiocaesium in the animal. Clay minerals from different sources have different binding capacities. It may be most effective to incorporate clay minerals into pelleted feeds at manufacture. This avoids loss of binder in feeding troughs
Requirements	
Specific equipment	None
Ancillary equipment	None
Utilities and infrastructure	Factory to incorporate clay minerals into pelleted feed rations during manufacture
Consumables	Clay minerals
Skills	Farmers would already possess the necessary skills
Budget	Expensive if incorporated into pelleted feed
Waste	
Amount and type	None
Impact	
Environmental	Effect of extracting large quantities of clay minerals on the landscape if quarry is not already in operation
Agricultural	Animal welfare issues associated with feeding atypically high quantities of clay minerals. Change in production status for organic farms
Social	May increase consumer confidence through effective management
Practical experience	
Evidence	Bentonite in conjunction with clean feed was used for reindeer in Sweden after Chernobyl. However, the cost was considered to be high relative to the additional 'effect' over clean feeding, so the practice was discontinued. Bentonite in concentrates was also used in Norway after Chernobyl for sheep, goats, cattle and reindeer but was substituted for AFCF from the second year due to higher effectiveness and easier handling of AFCF
Key references	
	IAEA (2012) International Atomic Energy Authority Technical Report Series No 475, Guidelines for Remediation Strategies to Reduce the Radiological Consequences of Environmental Contamination. IAEA, Vienna, 2012

(continued)

Table A1 (continued)

14 Administer AFCF boli to ruminants	
Objective	To reduce activity concentrations of radiocaesium in meat to below Operational Intervention Levels (OILs)
Management option description	Slow release boli containing ammonium-ferric-hexacyano-ferrate (AFCF, Giese-salt), an effective radiocaesium binder, have been developed to reduce the gut uptake of radiocaesium by ruminants in agricultural and seminatural environments, where animals are infrequently handled. Boli are particularly favourable for infrequently handled free-grazing animals such as sheep. The boli are produced by compression of a mixture of AFCF, barite and wax. To ease swallowing, the boli are immersed in liquid paraffin prior to administration. The boli (normally 2–3) are inserted into the rumen and gradually release AFCF. The release rate of AFCF follows first-order kinetics. Boli are particularly suitable for free-grazing ruminants and can be administered when they are gathered for routine handling operations. Boli are administered to meat-producing animals 2–3 months prior to slaughter, and to dairy animals every 6–8 months. Boli are made in different sizes to suit different animals. Live monitoring prior to slaughtering provides reassurance to consumers that the boli are an effective option
Target	Primarily meat-producing ruminants. Potential for milk-producing animals, although more likely that addition of AFCF to concentrate ration would be used. The AFCF boli cannot be used for monogastric animals such as pigs
Targeted radionuclides	**Known applicability:** ^{134}Cs, ^{137}Cs
Scale of application	Distributed to all ruminants eating contaminated feed – especially suitable for free-grazing or infrequently handled animals
Time of application	Medium to long term (lack of established production facilities or stockpiles means that it is not a potential management option for application in the early phase)
Effectiveness	
Management option effectiveness	Up to 80% reduction in lamb meat and goat milk, and up to 70% reduction in cows' milk. Effectiveness can be variable depending upon time between administration and slaughter – a reduction of 50–65% over a period of 9–11 weeks can be expected for sheep administered 3 waxed boli
Factors influencing effectiveness of procedure	Concentration of AFCF and number of boli used. The presence of a wax coating on the boli increases the release period from 2 to 3 months. Time between boli administration and slaughter (or live monitoring) and biological half-life of radiocaesium in treated animal species It is possible that some animals may be missed and not administered boli. Marking treated animals (e.g. with lanolin-based marker fluids) may provide reassurance that animals have been treated. However, treated animals can still regurgitate boli
Requirements	
Specific equipment	For sheep, cows and goats, the farmer can administer by hand or adapt dosing guns used for other intra-ruminal devices. For reindeer, a specifically designed instrument is needed for placing the bolus in the rumen because of the reindeer's narrow oesophagus
Ancillary equipment	Corrals and fences will be needed if being administered in remote from farmstead in areas where animals would not normally be gathered and handled

(continued)

Table A1 (continued)

14 Administer AFCF boli to ruminants	
Utilities and infrastructure	Factory to manufacture AFCF boli. Currently there are no commercial facilities available
Consumables	Boli with AFCF. Liquid paraffin to ease swallowing
Skills	Farmer would have required skills with little additional training, although for reindeer a veterinarian may be required
Budget	Expensive in terms of manufacture of AFCF boli. Expensive if farmer has to gather animals. Expensive if veterinarian is required to administer boli
Waste	
Amount and type	None
Impact	
Environmental	None
Agricultural	Limited impact as conventional farming practices can be maintained. Animal welfare when administering boli. Impact on farms with organic status. Detailed toxicological studies have shown that AFCF has no adverse effects on animal or human health
Social	Acceptability to farmers, food industry and consumers of using an additional feed additive to remove contamination from the gut of livestock
Practical experience	
Evidence	Used in production systems in Norway following Chernobyl. Also, tested on a number of upland farms in UK, where the standard Norwegian sheep boli were found to be too large for hill lambs in these areas. Smaller boli were developed and tested; these required higher, AFCF content which caused integrity problems of the bolus
Key references	
	Nisbet AF and Woodman RFM (2000). Options for the Management of Chernobyl-restricted areas in England and Wales. J Env Radioact 51, 239–254 IAEA (2012) International Atomic Energy Authority Technical Report Series No 475, Guidelines for Remediation Strategies to Reduce the Radiological Consequences of Environmental Contamination. IAEA, Vienna, 2012

15 Distribute salt licks containing AFCF	
Objective	To reduce activity concentrations of radiocaesium in meat or milk of free-grazing animals to below Operational Intervention Levels (OILs)
Management option description	In salt-deficient areas, the intake of salt by grazing animals may be suboptimal, and salt licks are annually placed on pastures to supplement their intake. Ammonium-ferric-hexacyano-ferrate (AFCF, Giese-salt), an effective radiocaesium binder, can be added to such licks (at 2.5%) to reduce the uptake of radiocaesium in the animal's gut. Live monitoring prior to slaughtering can be a good supplement to control the effectiveness of the management option for each animal or a selection within a herd/flock
Target	Meat- and milk-producing animals
Targeted radionuclides	**Known applicability:** ^{134}Cs, ^{137}Cs

(continued)

Table A1 (continued)

15 Distribute salt licks containing AFCF	
Scale of application	Large
Time of application	Medium to long term
Effectiveness	
Management option effectiveness	Around 50% reduction in uptake of radiocaesium. However, there is considerable variation in effectiveness between animals within a given flock/herd (due to willingness to visit salt licks). One 10 kg salt lick is sufficient for 20 sheep over 3 months or for 20 dairy cows during 10 days
Factors influencing effectiveness of procedure	Only likely to be effective in areas where animals are salt deficient. In coastal areas the pastures will naturally contain sodium, and the animals are unlikely to utilise salt licks Biological half-life of animal Effective administration of the salt licks, spatial application rate and stocking density
Requirements	
Specific equipment	None
Ancillary equipment	None
Utilities and infrastructure	Salt lick distribution is an existing practice in areas where this management option would be effective Manufacturing plants willing to incorporate AFCF into their products
Consumables	Salt licks containing 2.5% AFCF
Skills	Existing animal husbandry practice. Some training/development in manufacturing plants making large quantities of AFCF salt licks
Budget	Inexpensive (increased costs of production of AFCF rather than standard salt licks – factor of 5)
Waste	
Amount and type	None
Impact	
Environmental	None
Agricultural	Can maintain the production of meat and milk without disrupting the normal farming practices. Possible change in status of organic farms
Social	Acceptability to farmers/herders, food industry and consumers from using an additional feed additive to reduce uptake from the gut of livestock
Practical experience	
Evidence	Widely used in Norway since 1989 and still in use for cows, sheep, goats and reindeer grazing unimproved pastures. Has proven effective, easily practicable and cheap Suggestion that more AFCF salt licks should have been distributed on reindeer pastures than were used in Norway post-Chernobyl (this would increase operator time and transport costs – helicopter and/or specialised vehicles potentially being required)
Key references	
	IAEA (2012) International Atomic Energy Authority Technical Report Series No 475, Guidelines for Remediation Strategies to Reduce the Radiological Consequences of Environmental Contamination. IAEA, Vienna, 2012

(continued)

Table A1 (continued)

16 Closure of air intake systems at food processing plant	
Objective	To reduce contamination of foodstuffs from unfiltered air used in processing
Management option description	In food industries relatively large volumes of air are used for drying and roasting. Outdoor air may be used directly or after purification with filters. Contamination of foodstuffs can be prevented by halting those processes at risk before and during the passage of the plume. Normal operation should be able to be resumed soon after the passage of the plume
Target	Industrial food processing of milk, meat, eggs and fish products
Targeted radionuclides	All radionuclides
Scale of application	Potentially large scale
Time of application	Pre-deposition phase, before the passage of the radioactive plume, and should therefore be implemented as soon as risk becomes apparent
Effectiveness	
Management option effectiveness	For batch processes that are completed and stopped before passage of the plume, the effectiveness should be close to 100% assuming that processing is not restarted until air concentrations are reduced to close to background levels
Factors influencing effectiveness of procedure	Sufficient time is needed to stop any existing processing prior to passage of the plume Minimal time is required if processes can be shut down via a central control panel. Closing air intakes of an industrial plant can be more complicated. A decision on implementation will have to consider the (potentially unknown) technical consequences of a sudden shutdown of some industrial processes
Requirements	
Specific equipment	None
Ancillary equipment	None
Utilities and infrastructure	Access to air intake systems in industrial buildings and facilities
Consumables	None for implementation. Air filters need to be disposed of after passage of the plume
Skills	Competent persons may have to be called on to implement the option out of hours
Budget	Inexpensive
Waste	
Amount and type	Filters in air ventilation systems will require disposal
Possible transport, treatment and storage routes	Landfill
Impact	
Environmental	None
Agricultural	None

(continued)

Table A1 (continued)

16 Closure of air intake systems at food processing plant	
Social	As the measure is preventative, with little risk to consumers, it is likely to help maintain public confidence in the safety of food products and promote trust in authorities
Practical experience	
Evidence	Limited
Key references	
	Valmari T, Rantavaara A and Hänninen R (2004). Transfer of radionuclides from outdoor air to foodstuffs under industrial processing during passage of radioactive plume. STUK-A 209, Helsinki: Radiation and Nuclear Safety Authority. 50pp. + appendix 1p. (in Finnish with English summary)

17 Decontamination of milk	
Objective	To remove contamination from milk and return this milk to the food chain
Management option description	Techniques are available for removing radionuclides from milk on a large scale; these include magnetic separation, ion exchange, electrodialysis and ultrafiltration. A relatively new method, 'MAG*SEP^{SM}', uses specially coated magnetic particles that selectively remove radioactive contaminants from aqueous liquids, through selective adsorption and magnetic filtration
Target	Milk
Targeted radionuclides	**Known applicability**: ^{89}Sr, ^{90}Sr, ^{134}Cs, ^{137}Cs **Not applicable**: Radionuclides with short half-lives (e.g. ^{131}I)
Scale of application	Small to medium
Time of application	Medium to long term; decontamination equipment not stored for contingency purposes
Effectiveness	
Management option effectiveness	Ion exchange can result in the removal of up to 90% of the radionuclides Ultrafiltration can result in the removal of over 99% of caesium MAG*SEP^{SM} resins can remove over 99% of caesium Electrodialysis can result in the removal of up to 90% of the radionuclides
Factors influencing effectiveness of procedure	The decontamination process selected Radionuclide(s) present
Requirements	
Specific equipment	Decontamination unit – Lack of immediate availability (as of 2005 there are no decontamination units available for use outside the Ukraine) means that this measure is unlikely to be feasible in early phase. The manufacturers suggest that it would take up to 3 weeks for a separation unit to be set up to treat milk on an industrial scale
Ancillary equipment	None

(continued)

Table A1 (continued)

17 Decontamination of milk	
Utilities and infrastructure	Somewhere to site the decontamination unit, i.e. dairy
Consumables	Exchange resins/MAG*SEP^{SM} resins/ultrafiltration membranes/ electrodialysis membranes and salt solutions as required
Skills	Specific training in the techniques would be required for dairy personnel using the decontamination units. Specific training on the handling of waste
Budget	Expensive
Waste	
Amount and type	Used exchange resins/MAG*SEP^{SM} resins/ultrafiltration membranes/ electrodialysis membranes and salt solutions. Aqueous waste may also arise from regeneration of exchange resins and sorbents. Typically for ^{137}Cs 20 kg of resins are used to treat 100 batches of milk (each batch representing 1 metric tonne of milk). If radionuclide concentrations are well in excess of the OIL, waste stream may be very contaminated. Disposal of such materials would be subject to individual national regulations but might require licensing
Possible transport, treatment and storage routes	Disposal to landfill
Impact	
Environmental	Minimal
Agricultural	None
Social	Potential for rejection of the treated milk or decrease in market price depending on acceptability to consumers and retail trade Ion exchange and electrodialysis can result in adverse effects on the nutritional quality or organoleptic properties of the milk. MAG*SEP^{SM} does not adversely affect milk quality
Practical experience	
Evidence	MAG*SEP^{SM} used on an industrial scale to decontaminate milk in the Ukraine following the Chernobyl NRE: the nutritional quality, colour and smell were not affected
Key references	
	Long S, Pollard D, Cunningham JD, Astasheva NP, Donskaya GA and Labetsky EV (1995). The effects of food processing and direct decontamination techniques on the radionuclide content of foodstuffs: a literature review. Part 1: milk and milk products. Journal of Radioecology, 3,1, 15–30 Mercer J, Nisbet AF and Wilkins BT (2002). Management options for food production systems affected by a nuclear accident: 4 Emergency monitoring and processing of milk. NRPB-W15 Patel AA and Prasad SR (1993). Decontamination of radioactive milk – a review. International Journal of Radiation Biology, 63 (3), 405–412

(continued)

Table A1 (continued)

18 Dilution	
Objective	To provide milk with activity concentrations less than the Operational Intervention Levels (OILs)
Management option description	Contaminated milk may be mixed with uncontaminated milk in the appropriate proportions until the overall activity concentration in the bulk volume of milk is less than the maximum permitted level Good communication is required to set out the objectives and rationale of the option, using multiple channels (e.g. media, advisory centre, leaflets, internet). Possible advertising campaign highlighting environmental concerns/animal welfare issues if this management option is rejected in favour of disposal or slaughtering options
Target	Milk
Targeted radionuclides	All
Scale of application	Small to medium
Time of application	Early to medium term
Effectiveness	
Management option effectiveness	Can be highly effective in reducing volumes of milk requiring disposal. However, there would be no averted collective dose
Factors influencing effectiveness of procedure	Relative activity concentrations in contaminated and uncontaminated produce. Relative quantities of contaminated and uncontaminated produce. Extent to which supplies of either contaminated or uncontaminated produce are homogeneous This option would be most likely to be adopted when clean supplies were limited. Under such circumstances the amount of milk available as a diluent would also be limited
Requirements	
Specific equipment	None
Ancillary equipment	To allow optimal reduction in activity concentration of the final product sufficient numbers of containers may be required to allow the low and highly contaminated products to be stored separately until dilution took place
Utilities and infrastructure	A dairy. Communication channels
Consumables	Uncontaminated milk
Skills	The operators at the dairy and/or mill would have the necessary skills to carry out the dilution. Monitoring would be carried out by trained personnel
Budget	Inexpensive
Waste	
Amount and type	None
Impact	
Environmental	None
Agricultural	None
Social	Resistance from the dairy industry and retail trade. Possible rejection of the final product, decrease in market price. Potential for generating widespread mistrust

(continued)

Table A1 (continued)

18 Dilution	
Practical experience	
Evidence	Dilution was used in Valdres, Norway, where Chernobyl deposition was ~100 kBq/m^2. Some milk tankers collecting milk from this area were redirected to other dairies further away. In return, tankers from clean areas were sent to Valdres to dilute local supplies and so avoid the bulk milk exceeding the intervention limit. The redirection of milk tankers was a locally based decision that was not widely publicised
Key references	
	Woodman RFM, Nisbet AF and Penfold JSS (1997). Options for the management of foodstuffs contaminated as a result of a nuclear accident. NRPB-R295

19 Local provision of monitoring equipment	
Objective	To provide the general public or those with small holdings (backyard production) access to equipment or facilities to allow screening of feedstuffs or animal products for radioactivity content to make an informed choice about whether or not feedstuffs can be given to livestock or animal products can enter the food chain
Management option description	Establish an accredited monitoring service (fixed or mobile) at the local level to enable checks to be made on radionuclide content of animal feedstuffs and animal products
Target	Animal feedstuffs that might be contaminated. Animal products such as milk, meat and eggs
Targeted radionuclides	**Known applicability:** ^{131}I, ^{134}Cs, ^{137}Cs **Not applicable**: Radionuclides with no effective photon emissions (i.e. beta and alpha emitters, e.g. ^{90}Sr) and radionuclides with low photon energies (e.g. ^{239}Pu and ^{241}Am)
Scale of application	Small or medium scale. Areas where food is produced on a small scale (backyard production)
Time of application	Early to long term. Consumption of wild foodstuffs is likely to be restricted in the early phase until appropriate monitoring equipment is available
Effectiveness	
Management option effectiveness	This management option does not remove the contamination but is potentially highly effective for dose reduction by identifying contaminated feed and products. Decisions required
Factors influencing effectiveness of procedure	Time taken to distribute calibrated equipment and provide training may preclude the use of this management option for radionuclides with comparatively short half-lives Decisions on whether to exclude contaminated feed from animal diet. Decision on whether to dispose of contaminated animal products, rather than placing them in the food chain
Requirements	
Specific equipment	Spectrometry systems for the determination of gamma-ray-emitting radionuclides in foodstuffs

(continued)

Table A1 (continued)

19 Local provision of monitoring equipment	
Ancillary equipment	Data recording equipment
Utilities and infrastructure	Transport, distribution and co-ordination of monitoring equipment or service. Trained personnel to interpret and explain results to members of public and farmers
Consumables	Sample containers
Skills	Knowledge of radioanalytical and radiochemical methods; teaching for education and training of public (e.g. in use of counting equipment)
Budget	Expensive (provision of monitoring equipment and trained staff, plus potential disposal costs for contaminated foods)
Waste	
Amount and type	Feedstuffs and animal products that are contaminated to unacceptable levels will require disposal
Possible transport, treatment and storage routes	Landfill
Impact	
Environmental	None
Agricultural	Rejection of some foodstuffs may disrupt local practices
Social	Disruption of traditional food production. Potential for contaminated foodstuffs to enter black market
Practical experience	
Evidence	A similar scheme has worked successfully in the contaminated villages of Belarus for milk and mushrooms (Hériard Dubreuil et al., 1999)
Key references	
	Hériard Dubreuil GF, Lochard J, Girard P, Guyonnet JF, Le Cardinal G, Lepicard S, Livolsi P, Monroy M, Ollagon H, Pena-Vega A, Pupin V, Rigby J, Rolevitch I and Schneider T (1999). Chernobyl post-NRE management: the ETHOS project. *Health Phys* **77**, 361–372

20 Processing of milk for consumption	
Objective	To produce milk products with activity concentrations less than Operational Intervention Levels (OILs) from contaminated liquid milk that would be suitable for human consumption with or without a period of storage
Management option description	Processing would permit milk contaminated at levels above the OILs to be used for human consumption. Processing raw milk into butter and cheese may be used to reduce activity concentration of radiocaesium and radiostrontium to below the OIL. For ^{131}I and any other appropriate short-lived radionuclides, transformation into products with longer shelf-life such as cheese, UHT milk and canned goods is effective due to the short physical half-lives. Dialogue with milk industry and consumers is essential
Target	Milk

(continued)

Table A1 (continued)

20 Processing of milk for consumption	
Targeted radionuclides	**Known applicability**: ^{89}Sr, ^{90}Sr, ^{131}I, ^{134}Cs, ^{137}Cs
Scale of application	Small to medium scale
Time of application	Early to medium term
Effectiveness	
Management option effectiveness	**Radiocaesium and radioiodine.** Milk products prepared by isolating the fat and/or protein components from the aqueous fraction tend to be depleted in radiocaesium and radioiodine compared with raw milk. Examples are butter, cream, hard cheese, Greek "feta" cheese, cottage cheese, casein and whey protein concentrates **Radiostrontium.** Radiostrontium closely follows the behaviour of calcium. Hence, products such as cottage cheese, cream and butter, which are relatively low in calcium, tend to have low levels of radiostrontium, while high-calcium products such as skimmed milk and cheese have higher levels of radiostrontium. However, the transfer of radiostrontium during cheese making is affected by the method of coagulation used. If rennet coagulation is used, the transfer of radiostrontium to the cheese is usually increased. If acid coagulation is used, the transfer of radiostrontium to the cheese whey is increased The change in radionuclide content of a foodstuff due to processing may be assessed by considering **processing retention factor (Fr)** = total activity of the radionuclide in the processed food (Bq)/ total activity of the radionuclide in the raw material (Bq). Fr values are taken from Long et al. (1995) and IAEA (1994).

	^{131}I	^{134}Cs, ^{137}Cs	^{89}Sr, ^{90}Sr
	Fr	Fr	Fr
Milk powder	1.0	1.0	1.0
Cheese (rennet)	0.1–0.5	0.04–0.2	0.1–0.8
Cheese whey (rennet)	0.5–0.9	0.8–1.0	0.2–0.9
Cheese (acid)	0.2–0.3	0.1	0.04–0.1
Cheese whey (acid)	0.6–0.7	0.8–0.9	0.7–0.9
Cream	0.03–0.2	0.02–0.3	0.02–0.3
Butter	0.01–0.8	0.01–0.5	0.01–0.4
Skimmed milk	0.8–1.0	0.9–1.0	0.8–1.0
Cottage cheese (rennet)	0.05	0.01–0.1	0.03–0.3
Cottage cheese (acid)	0.2	0.1	0.1–0.2

	Effectiveness of processing into storable products such as UHT (ultrahigh temperature) milk will vary depending upon physical half-life and time stored prior to sale.
Factors influencing effectiveness of procedure	Radionuclide(s) present, fat content of milk, process selected
Requirements	
Specific equipment	Milk processing plant Special facilities may be required for milk products undergoing storage

(continued)

Table A1 (continued)

20 Processing of milk for consumption	
Ancillary equipment	Milk tankers
Utilities and infrastructure	Waste treatment facilities licensed to accept contaminated by-products
Consumables	Fuel for tankers
Skills	Operators at milk processing plants will have the required skills
Budget	Relatively inexpensive as processing equipment is already available. There may be additional costs of decontaminating equipment and for disposing of contaminated by-products. The option assumes that there is a market for the end product
Waste	
Amount and type	Percentage by mass of waste by-products generated in the production of various milk products for consumption: Cheese – 88% is cheese whey Butter – 52% is buttermilk Cream – 90% is skimmed milk Cottage cheese – 85% cottage cheese whey Milk powder/skimmed milk powder = no contaminated by-product (80–90% water) Contaminated water from washing and rinsing of tankers
Possible transport, treatment and storage routes	Dairy effluent plant and sewage treatment works
Impact	
Environmental	None provided by-products are disposed of appropriately
Agricultural	None
Social	Resistance from the dairy industry and retail trade. Possible rejection of the final product, decrease in market price. Potential for generating widespread mistrust
Practical experience	
Evidence	Milk above national intervention limits accepted for processing in the former Soviet Union (post-Chernobyl NRE)
Key references	
	Long S, Pollard D, Cunningham JD, Astasheva NP, Donskaya GA and Labetsky EV (1995). The effects of food processing and direct decontamination techniques on the radionuclide content of foodstuffs: a literature review. Part 1: milk and milk products. Journal of Radioecology, 3 (1), 15–30 Mercer J, Nisbet AF and Wilkins BT (2002). Management options for food production systems affected by a nuclear accident: 4 Emergency monitoring and processing of milk. NRPB-W15 Wilson L, Bottomley R and Sutton P (1988). Transfer of radioactive contamination from milk to commercial dairy products. Journal of the Society of Diary Technology, 41 (1), 10–13 IAEA (1994). Guidelines for agricultural countermeasures following an accidental release of radionuclides. Technical Report Series No. 363 IAEA (1994). Handbook of parameter values for the prediction of radionuclide transfer in temperate environments. Technical Report Series No. 364

(continued)

Table A1 (continued)

21 Product recall	
Objective	To prevent consumers eating contaminated food that may have entered the market
Management option description	Recall involves (i) advice to retailers to withdraw potentially contaminated products from sale and (ii) advice to members of the public to not consume specific products and to dispose of them or return them to the retail outlet for a refund. Provision of information about the recall and the reasons for it. Product recall would normally be carried out in conjunction with statutory restrictions on particular food products
Target	Food retailers and people who have purchased the affected products
Targeted radionuclides	All
Scale of application	Any
Time of application	Early phase, as soon as risk becomes apparent
Effectiveness	
Management option effectiveness	Very unlikely to be 100%. Cannot ensure that the recall message reaches all purchasers of affected batches. Some affected food may already have been consumed
Factors influencing effectiveness of procedure	Selection of suitable communication channels and clarity of information Difficulties tracing contaminated food that has been widely distributed the extent to which advice is followed (language and literacy issues)
Requirements	
Specific equipment	No specialist equipment is required to implement this option; however containers and temporary storage facilities may be needed for recalled food
Ancillary equipment	None
Utilities and infrastructure	Appropriate lines of communication Collection and disposal of recalled products
Consumables	Dependent on communication method (social media, retail websites, government websites, special interest groups (e.g. for contaminated infant formula or baby food), point-of-sale notices, newspaper and magazine adverts, television and radio (local and/or national), direct mailing (where possible and relevant)
Skills	Good communication with members of public is essential to prevent alarm
Budget	Recall is inexpensive but waste disposal could be expensive if done on large scale. Retailers will require compensation
Waste	
Amount and type	Depending on scale of the recall, it is possible that significant quantities of contaminated milk, meat and eggs may require disposal
Possible transport, treatment and storage routes	Milk may be spread on farmland, processed, biologically treated or disposed of to sea. Meat products may be disposed of by incineration or landfill. Ash from incineration would require disposal to landfill
Impact	
Environmental	None provided recalled products are disposed of appropriately

(continued)

Table A1 (continued)

21 Product recall	
Agricultural	None
Social	Potential for generating mistrust of food production systems or, conversely, possible increase in public confidence that the problem of contamination is being effectively managed
Practical experience	
Evidence	Product recalls are very common in some countries for non-radiological food scares

22 Raise intervention levels	
Objective	Raising intervention levels above Operational Intervention Levels to allow sale or use of foodstuffs
Management option description	Raising intervention levels in foodstuffs either because of the need to protect a particular producer/group or due to revision of dose-risk estimates. Usually most relevant for specialist or self-gathered or traditional foodstuffs. Likely to be controversial, so a good communication strategy will be essential
Target	Producers
Targeted radionuclides	**Known applicability**: ^{89}Sr, ^{90}Sr, ^{131}I, ^{134}Cs, ^{137}Cs, ^{239}Pu, ^{241}Am
Scale of application	Any
Time of application	Medium to long term (not relevant for the early phase as availability of measurements on which to base dose assessments is likely to be limited)
Effectiveness	
Management option effectiveness	Will lead to increased doses
Factors influencing effectiveness of procedure	Public/producers' perception and understanding of risks – likely to be closely linked to good communication and dialogue. Unlikely to be accepted without stakeholder consultation (producers, consumers, public)
Requirements	
Specific equipment	None
Ancillary equipment	None
Utilities and infrastructure	None
Consumables	Those associated with communication
Skills	Those associated with communication
Budget	Inexpensive. Costs will be associated with dissemination of information. Potential for compensation to food producers for possible reduced market value of foodstuffs
Waste	
Amount and type	None
Possible transport, treatment and storage routes	N/A

(continued)

Table A1 (continued)

22 Raise intervention levels	
Impact	
Environmental	Positive by maintaining traditional practices
Agricultural	Maintains ongoing agricultural practices
Social	Public confidence may be affected. Regional and cultural history will be decisive in determining acceptability of the option
Practical experience	
Evidence	Carried out in Scandinavia after Chernobyl (reindeer meat and freshwater fish). Good public acceptance in Norway (see Mehli et al., 2000) although some confusion over different levels within Europe reported from other countries. Intervention limits gradually reduced with time in former Soviet Union countries following the Chernobyl NRE
Key references	
	Mehli H, Skuterud L, Mosdøl A and Tønnessen A (2000). The impact of Chernobyl fallout on the Southern Saami reindeer herders in Norway in 1996. Health Physics, 79: 682–690

23 Restrict entry into the food chain	
Objective	To remove food that exceeds or potentially exceeds Operational Intervention Levels (OILs), from the food chain
Management option description	Milk, meat, eggs and fish with activity concentrations of radionuclides that exceed or potentially exceed Operational Intervention Levels (OILs) are withdrawn from sale. Requires a measurement programme to demonstrate compliance
Target	Milk, meat, eggs and fish. Also derived products from processing of these foodstuffs
Targeted radionuclides	All radionuclides
Scale of application	Large scale
Time of application	Predominantly early but possibly to long term
Effectiveness	
Management option effectiveness	Highly effective (up to 100%) at removing food containing radionuclides above OILs from the food chain. However, this option does not completely remove all contamination from the food chain as products with activity concentrations below the OILs can still enter the food chain
Factors influencing effectiveness of procedure	Availability of alternative supplies of food
Requirements	
Specific equipment	Monitoring and sampling equipment
Ancillary equipment	Additional containers and temporary storage facilities for waste may be needed
Utilities and infrastructure	Extensive monitoring and surveillance programme
Consumables	Any consumables required for sampling, monitoring and analysis work

(continued)

Table A1 (continued)

23 Restrict entry into the food chain	
Skills	Skilled personnel to carry out sampling, monitoring, analysis and data interpretation. Logistical experts to ensure maintenance of the food supply especially in early phase
Budget	Expensive (extensive monitoring required) – varies according to scale of restrictions
Waste	
Amount and type	Depending on size of area affected and duration of restrictions, it is possible that significant quantities of contaminated milk, meat and eggs may require disposal. Long-term restrictions may also lead to slaughter and disposal of livestock from dairy animals
Possible transport, treatment and storage routes	Milk may be spread on farmland, processed, biologically treated or disposed of to sea. Meat products may be disposed of by incineration, burning or burial. Ash from burning or incineration would require disposal to landfill
Impact	
Environmental	None
Agricultural	None, where restrictions are of short duration. If there are delays in restocking land, under-grazing of pasture could be a problem when animals return
Social	Extensive restrictions may lead to market shortages and disruption of farming and the food processing. Possible increase in price of food. Stigma associated with areas under food restrictions
Practical experience	
Evidence	Restrictions on meat occurred in many countries following the Chernobyl NRE. Similarly, the Japanese government stopped the distribution and sale of many contaminated food products including meat and fish following the Fukushima NRE
Key references	
	IAEA (2012) International Atomic Energy Authority Technical Report Series No 475, Guidelines for Remediation Strategies to Reduce the Radiological Consequences of Environmental Contamination. IAEA, Vienna, 2012

24 Salting of meat	
Objective	To produce meat products with activity concentrations less than Operational Intervention Levels from contaminated raw meat. Also applicable to contaminated fish
Management option description	Meat-producing livestock that have been slaughtered with activity concentrations of radiocaesium and radiostrontium above OILs may undergo salting either at commercial facilities or in the home. Meat pieces (200 g) are soaked in dilute NaCl brine (5%) using two successive treatments of 2 days each
Target	Meat or fish
Targeted radionuclides	**Known applicability:** ^{134}Cs, ^{137}Cs **Probable applicability**: ^{89}Sr, ^{90}Sr **Not applicable:** ^{239}Pu, ^{241}Am and radionuclides with short physical half-lives, e.g. ^{131}I

(continued)

Table A1 (continued)

24 Salting of meat	
Scale of application	Small to medium
Time of application	Medium to long term
Effectiveness	
Management option effectiveness	After soaking in salt solution, radiocaesium and radiostrontium contamination of meat may both be reduced by up to 80%
Factors influencing effectiveness of procedure	Size of the meat pieces treated – if large pieces, then a maximum reduction in radiocaesium contamination of 40–50% can be expected Concentration of salt solution and duration of treatment
Requirements	
Specific equipment	Food processing plant to carry out salting of meat
Ancillary equipment	Vehicles to transport contaminated meat to processing plant
Utilities and infrastructure	Waste treatment facilities for disposal of by-products
Consumables	Fuel for vehicles, additional salt
Skills	Operators at processing plants should have the required skills
Budget	Moderately expensive if new processes have to be set up. There may be additional costs of decontaminating equipment and for disposing of contaminated by-products. The option assumes that there is a market for the end product
Waste	
Amount and type	Large volumes of contaminated salt solution
Possible transport, treatment and storage routes	On-site treatment plants and sewage treatment works
Impact	
Environmental	None
Agricultural	None
Social	Resistance from the meat industry and retail trade. Possible rejection of the final product, decrease in market price. Disruption to the supply of meat to food industry and potential for market shortages. May impact public confidence Soaking meat in brine can affect its nutritional value removing water-soluble vitamins and water-soluble and salt-soluble proteins. Flavour of the meat may be adversely affected
Practical experience	
Evidence	Experimental only
Key references	
	Petaja E, Rantavaara A, Paakkola O and Puolanne E (1992). Reduction of radioactive caesium in meat and fish by soaking. Journal of Environmental Radioactivity, 16, 273–285 Long S, Pollard D, Cunningham JD, Astasheva NP, Donskaya GA and Labetsky EV (1995). The effects of food processing and direct decontamination techniques on the radionuclide content of foodstuffs: A literature review. Journal of Radioecology, 3, 1, 15–38

(continued)

Table A1 (continued)

25 Biological treatment of milk	
Objective	To reduce the mass of solids derived from contaminated milk requiring disposal
Management option description	Milk may be processed through aerobic (activated sludge or fixed-film systems) and anaerobic digestion (AD) facilities present in sewage treatment works (STWs) and dairy effluent plants (DEPs). In aerobic systems the provision of oxygen and bacteria accelerates processes that would naturally occur in oxygenated rivers. In anaerobic systems material is retained in an enclosed reactor at temperatures of 35–55 °C for a period of 10–30 days. These biological treatments accelerate a series of natural processes and significantly reduce the mass of solids for disposal and the biological oxygen demand of the effluent. Sludge and cake produced can be used as fertiliser and biogas for heating and electricity generation
Target	Contaminated milk
Targeted radionuclides	**Applicable:** ^{89}Sr, ^{90}Sr, ^{134}Cs, ^{137}Cs, ^{239}Pu and ^{241}Am
Scale of application	Small
Time of application	Early to late phase
Effectiveness	
Management option effectiveness	This management option does not remove the contamination but removes contaminated milk from the food chain
Factors influencing effectiveness of procedure	Dairy wastes at sewage treatment works cause problems due to the inadequate size of the plant and insufficient balancing (maximum holding capacity of one days average flow). STWs are not designed for the high BOD of dairy waste. Water companies usually insist that the fat content should not exceed 150 mg l^{-1} and pH should be between 6 and 9 and BOD between 300 and 600 mg l^{-1}. The optimum dry matter content for anaerobic digestion is 6–8%. To reduce raw milk's dry matter content to 6–8%, it has to be diluted with water to produce a 40% milk/60% water mixture Long residence time of milk in anaerobic reactor Capacity to treat contaminated milk depends on radiological impact of effluent, i.e. partitioning of radionuclides between effluent and sludge Willingness of STWs or DEPs to treat contaminated milk. Acceptability of disposal routes for sludge. Willingness of privately owned landfill sites and local populations to accept the wastes
Requirements	
Specific equipment	Biological treatment facility
Ancillary equipment	Vehicles for transport. Equipment for spreading sludge and cake
Utilities and infrastructure	Agricultural land, landfill and incinerators for sludge and cake disposal. Adequate storage space is required at the farm for sludge and cake prior to landspreading
Consumables	Fuel for transport

(continued)

Table A1 (continued)

25 Biological treatment of milk	
Skills	The necessary skills should be available at commercial facilities. Special attention must be given to the quantities of milk treated because of its potential to 'poison' the process because too much milk stops the digestion process The farmer will have experience of spreading wastes to land
Budget	Moderate (compensation to biological treatment facilities, transport companies, incineration and landfill operators for handling contaminated milk/sludge and for decontamination of equipment)
Waste	
Amount and type	**Anaerobic:** Typically, the volume of material is reduced by 40 to 60%, but it can be as high as 80%. Sludge can be treated further to produce a solid cake and liquid. The anaerobic digestion produces biogas, typically made up of 65% methane and 35% carbon dioxide, with conversion of solids to biogas ranging from 30 to 80% **Aerobic:** Sludge is produced, and the amounts depend on the micro-organisms present, BOD of milk, treatment method used, etc. Excess sludge represents 1%–5% of the volume of waste treated
Possible transport, treatment and storage routes	**Sludge and sludge cake** can be used in agriculture as fertilisers or sent to landfill or incineration for disposal. Sludge produced aerobically at a STW needs to be anaerobically treated in accordance with the 'Safe Sludge Matrix' before it can be spread on agricultural land **Liquid** generated during cake production is usually returned to the beginning of the treatment process (anaerobic treatment) or discharged to a water course (aerobic treatment) **Biogas** is normally used for process heating and electricity generation
Impact	
Environmental	Minimal provided guidelines are followed
Agricultural	Application of sludge or cake provides additional nutrients for crop uptake and could lead to reduced requirements for fertiliser. The cake also provides organic matter that improves the soil quality
Social	Willingness of farmers to accept sludge from biological treatment of milk. Resistance if the resulting sludge is applied to previously uncontaminated areas, or if the application restricts subsequent use, e.g. organic farming. Perception of causing additional contamination of the soil when slurry spread on farmland. Contamination of soil may restrict subsequent uses (e.g. organic farming) or generate stigma where sludge is spread on clean land
Practical experience	
Evidence	Biological treatment is a current practice at all sewage treatment works and dairy effluent plants. Disposal of raw milk to STWs has been carried out on a small scale. STWs are ubiquitous, whereas DEPs are only found in milk-producing area. DEPs treat large volumes of dilute milk processing wastes

(continued)

Table A1 (continued)

25 Biological treatment of milk	
Key references	
	Nisbet AF, Marchant JK, Woodman RFM, Wilkins BT and Mercer JA (2002). Management options for food production systems affected by a nuclear accident: (7) Biological treatment of contaminated milk. Chilton, NRPB-W38 Marshall KR and Harper WJ (1984). The Treatment of Wastes from the Dairy Industry. In Surveys in Industrial Wastewater Treatment. Barnes D, Forster CF and Hurdey SE (Eds). Pitman Publishing, London, 296–376 Wheatley AD (2000). Food and Wastewater. In Food Industry and the Environment in the European Union. Practical Issues and Cost Implications. 2nd Edition. Dalzell JM (Ed). Aspen Publishers Inc. Maryland

26 Burial of animal carcasses	
Objective	To dispose of animal carcasses following slaughter
Management option description	After slaughter animal carcasses may be disposed of in purpose-built burial pits, on-farm or at mass burial sites
Target	Meat- and milk-producing livestock
Targeted radionuclides	**Applicable:** ^{134}Cs, ^{137}Cs, ^{239}Pu, ^{241}Am **Not applicable**: Radionuclides with a high soil mobility as this may cause rapid movement into ground (e.g. ^{89}Sr, ^{90}Sr, ^{131}I)
Scale of application	Medium to large
Time of application	Early to late phase
Effectiveness	
Management option effectiveness	This management option does not remove the contamination but removes contaminated livestock from the food chain
Factors influencing effectiveness of procedure	Suitability and availability of land for burial pit (i.e. away from water sources and not on land with high water table), engineering of burial pit and maintenance of correct burial pit procedures On-farm burial site relies on the dispersal and dilution of animal leachate (fluids from carcasses) in the ground to protect water, so number of disposal sites is limited. Normally 8 tonnes of carcasses can be buried. This is equivalent to 16 adult cattle, 40 pigs or 100 sheep. More may be allowed in a crisis Mass burial site: Sewage treatment works (STWs) must have the capacity to treat the volumes of animal leachate produced. Time to construct mass burial sites. Transportation of carcasses to burial site Willingness of private landowners and local populations to accept carcasses for burial

(continued)

Table A1 (continued)

26 Burial of animal carcasses	
Requirements	
Specific equipment	Civil engineering equipment required to dig pit (e.g. bulldozers, JCBs), clay, geoclay liner and geocomposite liner to line mass burial pit, appropriate equipment to vent gas and collect animal leachate. Lamps to allow night working. All-purpose-built burial pits should ensure that carcasses remain permanently buried in such a way that carnivorous animals cannot gain access to them Ideally on-site treatment facilities to pretreat leachate and reduce biological strength before removal to sewage treatment works (either inland or coastal). Fencing to contain the site and prevent dumping of non-carcass material
Ancillary equipment	Transportation of carcasses to burial site and animal leachate to sewage treatment works
Utilities and infrastructure	Animal leachate has to be removed by tanker for treatment and disposal at sewage treatment works and on-site gas control measures On-site gas control measures
Consumables	Fuel for transportation of carcasses to burial pit and animal leachate to sewage treatment works
Skills	Engineers and construction workers to build burial pit
Budget	Expensive
Waste	
Amount and type	Animal leachate, e.g. body fluids from carcasses are released (about 0.1 m^3 per adult sheep and 1.0 m^3 per adult cow) within the first year, and gas
Possible transport, treatment and storage routes	Animal leachate has to be removed by tanker for treatment and disposal at sewage treatment works and on-site treatment of gas
Impact	
Environmental	Animal leachate may contain very high concentrations of ammonium (2000 mg l^{-1}), COD (100,000 mg l^{-1}) and potassium (3000 mg l^{-1}), sheep dip chemicals, barbiturates, disinfectants and pathogens. However, there is minimal risk of contamination of surface water and groundwater from leachate from correctly designed and managed purpose-built burial pits. In the early stages of decomposition, carcasses will release carbon dioxide and other gases such as methane, carbon monoxide and hydrogen sulphide There is a potential risk from carcasses awaiting disposal to contaminate private and public water supplies
Agricultural	Potential risk of land becoming blighted
Social	Disruption to farming and other related activities, e.g. tourism. Contamination of the soil may restrict subsequent uses (e.g. organic farming). Potential for dispute regarding selection of burial pit sites
Practical experience	
Evidence	Mass burial occurred in the UK to deal with foot and mouth infected animal carcasses where multiple pits each capable of holding 10,000–60,000 carcasses were constructed

(continued)

Table A1 (continued)

26 Burial of animal carcasses	
Key references	
	Department of Health (2001). Foot and Mouth Disease. Measures to Minimise Risk to Public Health from Slaughter and Disposal of Animals – Further Guidance. 24 April 2001 Environment Agency (2001). The Environmental Impact of the Foot and Mouth Disease Outbreak: An Interim Assessment. December 2001. Food Standards Agency (2002). Foot and Mouth disease. MAFF (2001). Guidance Note on the Disposal of Animal By-Products and Catering Waste. January 2001 Trevelyan GM, Tas MV, Varley EM and Hickman GAW (2001). The disposal of carcasses during the 2001 Foot and Mouth disease outbreak in the UK. Defra, FMD Joint Co-ordination Centre, Page Street, London, SW1P 4Q, UK

27 Burning of animal carcasess	
Objective	To dispose of animal carcasses following slaughter
Management option description	After slaughter, animal carcasses may be completely destroyed to ash, at sites suitable for burning
Target	Meat- or milk-producing livestock
Targeted radionuclides	**Applicable:** ^{89}Sr and ^{90}Sr (but are mobile in soil), ^{239}Pu, ^{241}Am **Not applicable**: Volatilisation of ^{131}I, ^{134}Cs and ^{137}Cs (as temperatures in excess of 400 °C) may occur
Scale of application	Medium to large
Time of application	Early to late phase
Effectiveness	
Management option effectiveness	This management option does not remove the contamination, but removes contaminated livestock from the food chain
Factors influencing effectiveness of procedure	Availability of suitable sites for burning and of burning materials. Quantity of carcasses Poorly constructed pyre can burn for several weeks
Requirements	
Specific equipment	Excavators for digging trenches. JCBs, forklift trucks and tractors with bucket loaders for moving fire ingredients and carcasses. Lamps to allow night working
Ancillary equipment	Vehicles for the transportation of carcasses to site for burning and to the ash disposal site Equipment to monitor air/water quality in area around burning site
Utilities and infrastructure	Burning site with good road network

(continued)

Table A1 (continued)

27 Burning of animal carcasess	
Consumables	To destroy 250 carcasses, the following are required: 250 railway sleepers, 250 bales of straw, 6250 kg of kindling wood, 50,750 kg of coal, 1 gallon of diesel oil per metre length of pyre
Skills	Continued supervision of burning
Budget	Expensive (excavation of burial site, fuel, operator time to supervise burning, monitoring)
Waste	
Amount and type	Ash – approximately 350 kg per animal
Possible transport, treatment and storage routes	Ash may be disposed of via burial in situ or transported to a fully instrumented landfill site
Impact	
Environmental	Short-term air quality and odour issues. Atmospheric emissions from pyres include gases, mineral dust, heavy metals, organic molecules and radionuclides. All of these are damaging to human and animal health and the environment and can enter the food chain downwind. Ash will contain radionuclides, heavy metals and hydrocarbons. A minimum distance of around 3 km should be left between pyres and housing Leachate from ash can produce ammonia, phosphorous and potassium. Therefore there is a risk of surface water and groundwater pollution from ash-associated contaminants, and to groundwater from fuels used There is a potential risk from carcasses awaiting burning to contaminate private and public water supplies. The risk will depend on state of decomposition
Agricultural	Ash has high concentrations of micro- and macronutrients that will fertilise the soil
Social	Disruption to farming and other related activities, e.g. tourism. Policing the carcass burning and averting growth of a black market in slaughtered animals. Potential for dispute regarding burning sites and selection of areas for ash disposal. Stigma associated with areas surrounding designated burning sites
Practical experience	
Evidence	Over 950 pyres were built in England and Wales during the foot and mouth disease (FMD) outbreak to control the spread of the disease. A limit of 1000 cattle per pyre was introduced during the outbreak though the Department of Health recommends smaller ones to reduce the amounts of air pollutants
Key references	
	Environment Agency (2001). The environmental impact of the foot and mouth disease outbreak: An interim assessment. December 2001. Environment Agency, Bristol, UK Trevelyan GM, Tas MV, Varley EM and Hickman GAW (2001). The Disposal of Carcasses during the 2001 Foot and Mouth Disease Outbreak in the UK. Defra, FMD Joint Co-ordination Centre, Page Street, London SW1P 4Q, UK

(continued)

Table A1 (continued)

28 Disposal of contaminated milk to sea	
Objective	To dispose of contaminated milk
Management option description	Contaminated milk may, in principle, be discharged to sea via outfalls of coolant water or liquid effluent at nuclear installations or via long sea outfalls at coastal sewage treatment works. Need for widespread dialogue to ascertain the acceptability of discharge to sea both nationally and internationally. Dialogue with the operators and regulators needs to be established well in advance. Potential need to facilitate widespread debate regarding the ethics and practice of disposal at sea. Requirement to monitor water quality in surrounding waterbody
Target	Contaminated milk
Targeted radionuclides	**Applicable:** ^{89}Sr, ^{90}Sr, ^{131}I, ^{134}Cs, ^{137}Cs **Not applicable:** ^{239}Pu, ^{241}Am
Scale of application	Potentially large scale
Time of application	Early to late phase
Effectiveness	
Management option effectiveness	This management option does not remove the contamination, but removes contaminated milk from the food chain
Factors influencing effectiveness of procedure	Ability to transport waste milk to discharge points and offload it easily. Limits on total BOD discharged by long sea outfalls that vary according to the degree of mixing of the receiving waterbody Compliance or resistance to the waste management option by operators, haulage companies and the public
Requirements	
Specific equipment	Large-capacity vehicles with specialised equipment and couplings for transport
Ancillary equipment	At some nuclear installations, pumps will be required to offload milk from tankers into holding pits
Utilities and infrastructure	Coolant water and liquid effluent outfalls at nuclear installations or long sea outfalls at sewage treatment works
Consumables	Fuel for transporting milk to outfall
Skills	Disposal of milk to sea will require preplanning, e.g. doing site-specific modelling to check environmental impact, liaison with nuclear or sewage plant operators The vehicle drivers and operators at the power stations and sewage works should have the necessary skills. However, the discharge of milk to sea is a non-standard practice that will require station managers to carry out a full risk assessment
Budget	Expensive (cost of tanker and fuel; time of drivers, operators at power stations/sewage works; decontamination of tankers; monitoring of water; etc.)
Waste	
Amount and type	No secondary waste
Impact	
Environmental	Effects of discharge on the dissolved oxygen content of the seawater should be small but must have been demonstrated in advance on a site-specific basis. In the worst case, dissolved oxygen content should return to ambient levels within about 17 days if 40 million litres are discharged over a 6-week period

(continued)

Table A1 (continued)

28 Disposal of contaminated milk to sea	
Agricultural	None
Social	Potential for dispute regarding selection of this waste disposal option. Stigma associated with areas where milk has been disposed of to sea, with potential impacts on tourism
Practical experience	
Evidence	Milk discharged to drains following Windscale fire
Key references	
	Wilkins BT, Woodman RFM, Nisbet AF and Mansfield PA (2001). Management options for food production systems affected by a nuclear accident. 5. Disposal of waste milk to sea. Chilton, NRPB-R323

29 Incineration	
Objective	To reduce volume of contaminated food products prior to disposal and to produce a stable end product
Management option description	Controlled burning of waste at high temperatures, typically around 900 °C. Organic components present in waste are released as exhaust gases, and mineral matter is left as a residual ash. The volume of the ash is about an order of magnitude less than the original waste; the corresponding reduction in terms of mass is about a factor of 3. The ash is typically disposed of to landfill A major disadvantage of incinerators is a low tolerance for non-combustible material that can be present in the inflowing material mix. This can be resolved through sorting material before it is sent to the facility
Target	Contaminated fish, rendered meat, eggs and milk powder (milk would require dewatering prior to incineration)
Targeted radionuclides	**Applicable**: ^{89}Sr, ^{90}Sr, ^{239}Pu, ^{241}Am **Not applicable**: ^{131}I, ^{134}Cs and ^{137}Cs will volatilise at 184 °C and 671 °C respectively
Scale of application	Medium to large. There may be limitations due to cost or capacity
Time of application	Early to late
Effectiveness	
Management option effectiveness	This management option does not remove the contamination but removes contaminated products from the food chain
Factors influencing effectiveness of procedure	Energy value, moisture content and combustibles content of the material affect the success of this procedure. In order to sustain combustion, the feedstock should have the following characteristics: energy value, minimum 6 MJ kg^{-1}; moisture content, maximum 35%; combustibles content, minimum 30% In addition, the operating temperature of incinerator, combustion conditions and physiochemical form of the radionuclides and the waste also affect this procedure. The operating temperature of the furnace must be maintained above 900 °C The majority of carcass incineration plants are not large enough to accommodate a whole bovine carcass

(continued)

Table A1 (continued)

29 Incineration	
Requirements	
Specific equipment	Commercial incinerators, on-farm incinerators and mobile air-curtain incinerators capable of disposing of mammalian carcasses
Ancillary equipment	Vehicles for transporting carcasses to incineration site and ash to landfill site
Utilities and infrastructure	If ash can't immediately be sent to landfill, it must be safely stored
Consumables	Fuel for transporting carcasses to incineration site and to run incinerator. Mobile air-curtain incinerators only work effectively when fed with dry seasoned timber
Skills	Trained personnel will be available at incineration facilities. Operators require information on the incineration of contaminated material
Budget	Expensive
Waste	
Amount and type	Ash. The volume of ash produced is usually 10% of the original material, and the mass is reduced to 25–30% of the original material. The ash is likely to have a higher activity concentration than the original material. This is due to the volume of original material being greatly reduced and the majority of radionuclides being retained in the ash, with some activity being released in the flue gases. Ash may be fully immobilised by conditioning in cement or other suitable matrix prior to disposal
Possible transport, treatment and storage routes	Ash from commercial incinerators must be disposed of to landfill. Ash from air-curtain and on-farm incinerators can be buried on site providing there is no possibility of groundwater and surface water contamination. Otherwise it must be collected, stored and sent to landfill
Impact	
Environmental	Atmospheric emissions from incineration include gases; mineral dust; heavy metals; and organic molecules. All of these are damaging to human and animal health and the environment. However, the amounts discharged have been significantly (and continue to be) reduced due to advances in incinerator and flue gas treatment technologies. Radionuclides released during incineration may be taken up into the food chain by animals grazing on grass nearby. Possible risk of pollution to soil, surface waters and groundwaters from ash-associated contaminants
Agricultural	Ash has high concentrations of micro- and macronutrients that will fertilise the soil
Social	Possible local opposition due to perception that radionuclides will be released to atmosphere
Practical experience	
Evidence	Some BSE-infected cattle, specified risk material (SRM) and Over Thirty Month Scheme (OTMS) cattle were incinerated during the foot and mouth disease (FMD) crisis in the UK, although due to the high costs and the limited capacity of incineration, most were disposed of by alternative methods. Incineration is frequently used as a disposal route for household waste, as landfill space becomes less available

(continued)

Table A1 (continued)

29 Incineration	
Key references	
	Bontoux L (1999). The Incineration of Waste in Europe: Issues and Perspectives, IPTS, March 1999 IAEA (2011) Final Report of the International mission on Remediation of Large Contaminated Areas Off-Site the Fukushima Daiichi NPP 7–15 October 2011, Japan, IAEA NE/NEFW/2011, 15/11/2011 IAEA (2014) The follow-up IAEA International Mission on Remediation of Large Contaminated Areas Off-Site the Fukushima Daiichi Nuclear Power Plant. Tokyo and Fukushima Prefecture, Japan. 14–21 October 2013. Final report 23/01/2014 Stanners D and Bourdeau P (Eds) (1995). Europe's Environment: The Dobris Assessment – An overview. European Environment Agency, Copenhagen Woodman RFM, Nisbet AF and Penfold JSS (1997). Options for the management of foodstuffs contaminated as a result of a nuclear accident. Chilton, NRPB-R295

30 Landfill	
Objective	To dispose of contaminated food products before or after volume reduction techniques
Management option description	Organic material can be disposed of to fully engineered landfill sites. These have clay or membrane liners and collection systems designed to contain leachates and landfill gas
Target	Rendered meat, eggs, milk powder, fish
Targeted radionuclides	**Applicable:** ^{134}Cs, ^{137}Cs, **Not applicable**: Radionuclides with high soil mobility (e.g. ^{89}Sr, ^{90}Sr, ^{131}I). Radionuclides with short half-lives (e.g. ^{131}I)
Scale of application	Large
Time of application	Early to late phase
Effectiveness	
Management option effectiveness	This management option does not remove the contamination, but removes contaminated products from the food chain
Factors influencing effectiveness of procedure	Large quantities of putrescible wastes can cause instability and uneven settlement in a landfill. Therefore the maximum proportion of putrescible wastes which could practicably be disposed of to landfill is estimated to be 50% by weight of the inventory. Putrescible waste must be thoroughly mixed with inert wastes to provide a suitable medium to allow continuation of normal landfill operations. Future management of landfills may further restrict quantities of putrescible wastes admitted. Disposal must be to a fully engineered sanitary landfill licensed to accept putrescible waste. Maintenance of landfill procedures Willingness of privately owned landfill sites and local populations to accept the wastes

(continued)

Table A1 (continued)

30 Landfill	
Requirements	
Specific equipment	Landfill site
Ancillary equipment	Vehicles for transport of food products, compost, soil and ash to landfill
Utilities and infrastructure	Appropriate transport network
Consumables	Fuel for transport of food products, compost, soil and ash to landfill
Skills	At landfill sites the necessary skills will be available
Budget	Expensive
Waste	
Amount and type	Leachate, landfill gas (methane and carbon dioxide)
Possible transport, treatment and storage routes	Leachate treatment may involve on-site pretreatment including aeration, biodegradation or reed bed filtration. The treated leachate can be discharged to a sewer or directly tankered away for further treatment at a sewage treatment works (STWs). It can also be discharged to waterways provided the relevant discharge authorisations are held Landfill gas is usually managed either by a pumping system with passive venting or flaring or by a pumping system with a condensation system to remove moisture and permit use of gas for heating or electricity generation
Impact	
Environmental	In a fully engineered site, leachate will be collected and disposed of via an appropriate route, so environmental impact should be minimised. A high proportion of food wastes in a landfill would provide conditions for maximum gas production – both methane and carbon dioxide are greenhouse gases that contribute to global climate change. Unless landfill gas is used for electricity generation, landfilling of organic wastes will not result in energy or nutrient recovery
Agricultural	None
Social	Possible local opposition about disposal of contaminated produce to landfill
Practical experience	
Evidence	Landfill is a current practice
Key references	
	Nakano M. and Yong RN (2013). Overview of rehabilitation schemes for farmlands contaminated with radioactive cesium released from Fukushima power plant. Engineering Geol 2013; 155:87–93 Woodman RFM, Nisbet AF and Penfold JSS (1997). Options for the management of foodstuffs contaminated as a result of a nuclear accident. Chilton, NRPB-R295

(continued)

Table A1 (continued)

31 Landspreading of milk and/or slurry	
Objective	To dispose of contaminated milk and/or slurry
Management option description	Some agricultural land is potentially suitable for the spreading of milk, either in conjunction with slurry or diluted with water. The spreading of slurry is a normal agricultural practice. In the event of a NRE, contaminated milk and slurry would be landspread in situ
Target	Contaminated milk and/or contaminated slurry
Targeted radionuclides	**Applicable:** ^{89}Sr, ^{90}Sr, ^{131}I, ^{134}Cs, ^{137}Cs, ^{239}Pu and ^{241}Am
Scale of application	Large-scale application on most farms that stock dairy herds. Application may be more restricted on farms stocking alpine sheep and goats
Time of application	Early to medium term. Landspreading milk is highly seasonal, because of the danger of pollution when fields are waterlogged or frozen. Under such circumstances it is possible to store the milk in slurry tanks, if space is available; spreading may then be carried out at a later date
Effectiveness	
Management option effectiveness	This management option does not remove the contamination, but removes contaminated products from the food chain
Factors influencing effectiveness of procedure	Land available for landspreading. Soil type. Storage space in slurry tank. Environmental conditions on farm. Radionuclide content of the milk or slurry Degree to which landspreading diverges from common practice will affect willingness of farmers to implement this option. Status of the land Milk should not be spread on land with a high risk of run-off or near to any water courses, and should be diluted with the same volume of water or slurry. The amount of diluted milk spread at any one time should not exceed 50 m^3 ha^{-1} $year^{-1}$, and at least 3 weeks should be left between each application to reduce surface sealing. On bare land the soil should be lightly cultivated after spreading to quickly mix the waste
Requirements	
Specific equipment	Slurry transport and distribution systems (usually available on farms)
Ancillary equipment	Slurry storage tanks (usually available on farm)
Utilities and infrastructure	None
Consumables	Fuel
Skills	Farmers would possess the necessary skills as landspreading is an existing practice
Budget	Inexpensive
Waste	
Amount and type	No secondary waste produced
Impact	
Environmental	Inappropriate disposal of milk to land could lead to pollution of water courses
Agricultural	Additional nutrients provided for crop uptake which could lead to reduced requirements for fertiliser

(continued)

Table A1 (continued)

31 Landspreading of milk and/or slurry	
Social	Perception of causing additional contamination of the soil if milk or slurry is spread on farmland. Willingness of farmer to carry out landspreading if this is not usual practice
Practical experience	
Evidence	Landspreading of milk is carried out on a small scale when farmers are over quota or there is evidence of microbiological contamination. It has not, however, been carried out on a large scale in the past
Key references	
	Marchant JK and Nisbet AF (2002). Management options for food production systems affected by a nuclear accident. 6. Landspreading as a waste disposal option for contaminated milk. Chilton, NRPB-W11

32 Processing and long-term storage	
Objective	To convert contaminated milk into a more stable end product for storage and subsequent disposal
Management option description	Milk processing facilities may be used to produce milk products that are suitable for storage and subsequent disposal. This would give the authorities additional time in which to consider disposal options. The most effective and straightforward option is the processing of liquid milk into whole milk powder
Target	Milk
Targeted radionuclides	**Applicable:** ^{89}Sr, ^{90}Sr, ^{131}I, ^{134}Cs, ^{137}Cs, ^{239}Pu and ^{241}Am
Scale of application	Medium to large
Time of application	Early to medium phase
Effectiveness	
Management option effectiveness	This management option does not remove the contamination, but removes contaminated products from the food chain
Factors influencing effectiveness of procedure	Availability and capacity of facilities for processing Availability of storage facilities and subsequent disposal routes
Requirements	
Specific equipment	Milk processing plant with freeze-drier
Ancillary equipment	Milk tankers
Utilities and infrastructure	Storage facilities for milk powder
Consumables	Fuel for tankers
Skills	Operatives at milk processing plants will have the required skills
Budget	Expensive, depending on transport distance, length of storage time, disposal route and costs for decontamination
Waste	
Amount and type	Milk powder. Contaminated water from washing and rinsing of tankers. Water extracted in production of milk powder is uncontaminated and does not require special disposal

(continued)

Table A1 (continued)

32 Processing and long-term storage	
Possible transport, treatment and storage routes	Milk powder can be disposed of to landfill. The stability of milk powder permits a period of storage (i.e. supervised warehouse) in advance of a suitable disposal route being found. Disposal of contaminated washings can be made to dairy effluent plants or sewage treatment works. Disposal of processing wastes would be subject to individual national regulations and may require licensing
Impact	
Environmental	Minimal provided milk powder is disposed of properly
Agricultural	None
Social	Resistance to allowing contaminated milk into dairies because retailers and consumers would not have the confidence that the plant could be put back to normal operation after treatment has taken place, without the risk of contaminating milk and milk products subsequently produced
Practical experience	
Evidence	Processing of milk to whole milk powder is a current practice
Key references	
	Long S, Pollard D, Cunningham JD, Astasheva NP, Donskaya GA and Labetsky EV (1995). The effects of food processing and direct decontamination techniques on the radionuclide content of foodstuffs: a literature review. Part 1: milk and milk products. *J Radioecol* **3** (1), 15–30 Mercer J, Nisbet AF and Wilkins BT (2002). Management options for food production systems affected by a nuclear accident: 4 Emergency monitoring and processing of milk. Chilton, NRPB-W15

33 Rendering	
Objective	To reduce volume of contaminated carcasses prior to disposal
Management option description	Animal carcasses may be sent to licensed rendering plants and reduced to tallow, meat and bonemeal (MBM), condensate (the condensed steam produced from boiling off the water from the rendering process) and blood. These products require subsequent disposal to landfill, incineration and wastewater treatment plant
Target	Meat- and milk-producing livestock
Targeted radionuclides	**Applicable:** ^{89}Sr, ^{90}Sr, ^{134}Cs, ^{137}Cs, ^{239}Pu and ^{241}Am **Not applicable**: Radionuclides with short half-lives (e.g. ^{131}I)
Scale of application	Medium to large
Time of application	Early to late phase
Effectiveness	
Management option effectiveness	This management option does not remove the contamination but removes contaminated products from the food chain
Factors influencing effectiveness of procedure	The availability and capacity of rendering plants to cope with large numbers of livestock carcasses at any one time. The reduction of the carcasses to tallow and meat and bonemeal (MBM) is dependent on temperature, time and pressure combinations at each facility

(continued)

Table A1 (continued)

33 Rendering	
Requirements	
Specific equipment	Rendering plants suitable for disposal of mammalian carcasses
Ancillary equipment	Transportation of carcasses from farm to rendering plant and waste products to landfill or incineration and wastewater treatment plant
Utilities and infrastructure	Disposal route for waste products, e.g. landfill, incineration, wastewater treatment
Consumables	Fuel for transportation of carcasses and waste products
Skills	Rendering operators should have the necessary skills
Budget	Expensive when carried out on a large scale
Waste	
Amount and type	When a whole carcass is rendered, the volume is reduced by 12%. Generally, this is made up of 60% MBM and 40% tallow. Upon incineration this is reduced further. Between 100 and 150 kg ash is produced per tonne of carcass MBM is a dust-like end product containing 60–65% protein, and tallow is solid hard fat
Possible transport, treatment and storage routes	Tallow and MBM may be incinerated (generating between 100 and 150 kg ash per tonne of carcass) and/or sent to licensed commercial landfill. Condensate has to be treated on site or at a wastewater treatment plant to produce clean water and sludge
Impact	
Environmental	Minimal from rendering itself. Rendering is the preferred method of whole carcass disposal as it has the least disposal hazards associated with it
Agricultural	None
Social	Minimal
Practical experience	
Evidence	Rendering was the preferred option for disposing of livestock during the foot and mouth disease (FMD) outbreak in the UK, although capacity was a limiting factor at the peak of the outbreak. Therefore, incineration, burial and burning disposal methods were also used. Rendering waste products were disposed of by incineration and landfill, depending on the rendering process used and age of cattle
Key references	
	MAFF (2001). Guidance Note on the Disposal of Animal By-Products and Catering Waste. January 2001 Trevelyan GM, Tas MV, Varley EM and Hickman GAW (2001). The disposal of carcasses during the 2001 Foot and Mouth disease outbreak in the UK. Defra, FMD Joint Co-ordination Centre, Page Street, London, SW1P 4Q, UK

Annex B: Worked Examples to Illustrate Decision-Aiding Framework

Anne Nisbet

Several hypothetical work examples have been developed to help illustrate how the decision-aiding framework can be used to select and combine options in the development of a management strategy. The examples are as follows:

- Example 1: Strategy for iodine contamination of intensive milk production (Table B1)
- Example 2: Strategy for caesium contamination in free-ranging lamb (Table B2)
- Example 3: Strategy for iodine and caesium contamination of poultry (Table B3)

The examples take users, in a very general way, through the main decision steps and the types of issues that they would need to address in the development of a recovery strategy. It is important to note that the worked examples provided are only illustrative. They have been included solely to support training in the use of the decision framework. The worked examples should not be used as definitive solutions to the contamination scenario selected.

Table B1 Worked example to illustrate a strategy for iodine contamination of milk (intensive production)

Radionuclide: ^{131}I
Product: Milk (several million litres, likely to exceed OIL without intervention)
Time of year: End of growing season
Type of land: Coastal lowland pasture (intensive production), Western Europe
Duration that OILs are exceeded: 60 days

Step	Action
1	**Identify one or more production systems that are likely to be/have been contaminated**
	It is milk production systems that have been affected. Management options are required for producing clean milk in the contaminated area as well as for disposing of contaminated milk above the OIL. These options will have to be in place for a period of up to 60 days
2	**Refer to selection table for specific production systems**
	Table 6.2 provides a list of all of the applicable management options for milk, including those for waste disposal. There are 11 options for live animals, 8 options for milk and 5 options for disposal. Of these, raising intervention levels (for protected lifestyles) and local provision of monitoring equipment (backyard production) are not appropriate for this intensive milk production scenario. Natural attenuation and monitoring can also be eliminated as some form of intervention is required to prevent several million litres of contaminated milk being produced

(continued)

Table B1 (continued)

<table>
<tr><td>3</td><td colspan="2">Refer to look-up tables showing applicability of management options, including those for waste disposal, for the radionuclide being considered</td></tr>
<tr><td></td><td colspan="2">Tables 6.4 (management options) and 6.5 (waste disposal options) provide information on the applicability of options for ^{131}I
Eight of the remaining management options identified in Table 6.2 can be eliminated on the basis of:
(i) Being specific for either Cs or Group II elements of the periodic table (i.e. addition of AFCF, calcium or clay minerals to feed; administration of AFCF boli; distribution of AFCF salt licks)
(ii) Requiring relatively long timescales for implementation and therefore inappropriate for radionuclides with short half-lives such as ^{131}I (i.e. selective grazing; select alternative land use; slaughtering of livestock; suppression of lactation)
A further waste disposal option (incineration) could be eliminated on the basis that ^{131}I would volatilise (and potentially be released to the environment) below the operating temperature of the process. At this stage, the following management options still need to be considered:</td></tr>
<tr><td></td><td><u>Live animals</u>
Clean feeding
Short-term sheltering
<u>Animal products</u>
Close air intake at processing plant
Dilution
Processing and storage for consumption
Product recall
Restrict entry into food chain</td><td><u>Disposal of milk</u>
Biological treatment of milk
Disposal of milk to sea
Landspreading of milk
Processing and long-term storage</td></tr>
<tr><td>4</td><td colspan="2">Refer to look-up table showing checklist of major constraints for each management option, including those for waste disposal</td></tr>
<tr><td></td><td colspan="2">Table 6.6 provides information on the key constraints for each option
Options to be implemented before arrival of the plume (i.e. short-term sheltering of dairy animals, closing air intake systems at processing factories) depend on the period of notification given. For most foreseeable future NREs, some form of early notification of a possible release would be expected. This makes the implementation of pre-deposition options more likely, especially at increasing distances from the site of the NRE. Constraints such as availability of suitable housing and supplies of alternative clean feeds for the short-term sheltering and subsequent clean feeding of livestock are unlikely to be significant in the autumn, as stored clean feed, harvested earlier in the year, would be available. Restrictions on the entry of milk into the food chain are based on statutory food restriction orders and will be legally binding, irrespective of any constraints. Where there is uncertainty that contaminated milk products may have entered the food chain before restrictions had been put in place, product recall is a possible option; both these options require plans for subsequent management of waste milk. Dilution of contaminated milk with clean supplies, and the processing and storage of milk products prior to consumption, while being technically feasible, may undermine consumer confidence
In terms of disposal options, biological treatment facilities have very limited capacity for milk and would not be able to provide a major disposal route in this particular scenario. Furthermore, water utilities may oppose entry of contaminated milk to their sites. Disposal of contaminated milk to sea via long sea outfalls may be possible as a last resort option requiring authorisation from the relevant environmental regulator. For milk held on the farm, landspreading of milk is possible according to the suitability of land. An option that 'buys time' is the processing of milk into powder and its storage for a period until a suitable disposal route is found. The requisitioning of such facilities is likely to be very expensive
At this stage, the following management options still need to be considered:</td></tr>
</table>

(continued)

Table B1 (continued)

<table>
<tr><td></td><td><u>Live animals</u>
Clean feeding
Short-term sheltering
<u>Animal products</u>
Close air intake at processing plant
Product recall
Restrict entry into food chain</td><td><u>Disposal of milk</u>
Disposal of milk to sea
Landspreading of milk
Processing and long-term storage</td></tr>
<tr><td>5</td><td colspan="2">Refer to look-up table showing effectiveness of management options</td></tr>
<tr><td></td><td colspan="2">Table 6.7 provides information on effectiveness. This clearly shows that all of the remaining options are highly effective and should produce milk or processed milk products with activity concentrations of ^{131}I less than the OIL</td></tr>
<tr><td>6</td><td colspan="2">Refer to look-up tables showing management options that incur an additional dose to those involved in their implementation either directly or through the management of any secondary wastes produced</td></tr>
<tr><td></td><td colspan="2">Tables 6.8 and 6.9 provide information on doses and waste production from the implementation of management options
Clearly the placing of restrictions on the entry of milk into the food chain and product recall generates waste, the management of which leads to additional doses to those carrying out disposal. Clean feeding of housed dairy livestock can incur small incremental doses to the farmer from carrying out a grassland management programme while the animals are indoors. This involves cutting and disposing of contaminated grass before animals are returned to pasture. Waste in the form of contaminated slurry may be generated by housed animals during their period of clean feeding but only if the animals had previously been grazing contaminated pasture. The collection and disposal of this waste incurs a further small incremental dose to the farmer
Disposal of milk to sea and the landspreading of milk are options that dilute and disperse ^{131}I, which reduce magnitude of individual doses received by members of the public. In contrast, processing (into a dried form) and long-term storage, concentrates and contains the contamination, which is likely to give rise to higher individual doses to those handling the by-products. A dose assessment should be carried out if this option is selected</td></tr>
<tr><td>7</td><td colspan="2">Refer to individual datasheets (Annex A) for all options remaining in the selection table, and note any further constraints</td></tr>
<tr><td></td><td colspan="2">This step involves a detailed analysis of all remaining options by careful consideration of the relevant datasheets. It can only be done on a site-specific basis and in close consultation with local stakeholders to take into account local circumstances</td></tr>
<tr><td>8</td><td colspan="2">Based on Steps 1–7, select and combine options that should be considered as part of the recovery strategy</td></tr>
<tr><td></td><td colspan="2">Options for producing clean milk/maintaining milk production
Pre-deposition phase: Short-term sheltering of dairy animals and closing air intake systems at milk processing plants, both options, assume adequate notification of release is given. The sheltering of dairy animals can be extended into the urgent and early phases and combined with clean feeding
Urgent–early phase: Restrict entry of milk into food chain; product recall; provide housing and clean feed until levels of ^{131}I in pasture decrease (around 60 days)
Note: The implementation of a clean feeding programme in the early phase should reduce the quantities of contaminated milk requiring disposal to manageable levels
Options for disposing of waste
For contaminated milk held on the farm: Landspreading of milk assuming soil conditions are suitable, making use of storage capacity in slurry tanks
For milk already collected or when landspreading is inappropriate, consider disposal to sea via a long sea outfall with authorisation from environmental regulator. Otherwise, investigate the requisitioning of a processing plant to convert milk into powder for storage and subsequent disposal. Carry out assessment of incremental doses to workers at the plant</td></tr>
</table>

Table B2 Worked example to illustrate a strategy for caesium contamination of lamb (extensive production)

Radionuclide: ^{134}Cs, ^{137}Cs
Product: Lamb (several thousands of sheep, will exceed OILs without intervention)
Time of year: Start of growing season
Type of land: A national park with upland organic soils (extensive production), Western Europe
Duration that OILs are exceeded: Predicted to be for several decades

Step	Action
1	**Identify one or more production systems that are likely to be/have been contaminated**
	It is meat production systems that have been affected. Management options are required for producing meat with activity concentrations below the OILs. Due to the organic nature of the soils leading to sustained availability of ^{134}Cs and ^{137}Cs, these options will have to be in place for a period of up to several decades
2	**Refer to selection table for specific production systems**
	Table 6.3 provides a list of management options for all types of meat production, including disposal of contaminated meat. Of these, change in hunting season, manipulating slaughter times, use of additives in feed and provision of monitoring equipment are not appropriate for extensively managed sheep production. Furthermore, natural attenuation and monitoring is not applicable in a situation where sheep meat is predicted to be contaminated for decades. Therefore, there are 7 options for live animals, 5 options for meat products and 5 options for disposal. These are the management options that still need to be considered:

Live animals: Change in husbandry	Animal products
Clean feeding	Close air intake at processing plant
Live monitoring	Product recall
Select alternative land use	Raise intervention levels
Selective grazing	Restrict entry into food chain
Slaughtering (culling) of livestock	Salting of meat
Live animals: Use of additives	Disposal of meat
Administration of AFCF boli to ruminants	Burial
Distribution of AFCF salt licks	Burning
	Incineration
	Landfill
	Rendering

Step	Action
3	**Refer to look-up tables showing applicability of management options, including those for waste disposal, for the radionuclide being considered**
	Tables 6.4 and 6.5 provide information on the applicability of options for ^{134}Cs and ^{137}Cs Two options for disposal of contaminated meat in Table 6.3 can be eliminated on the basis that ^{134}Cs and ^{137}Cs would volatilise during incineration or when carcasses are burned, resulting in release of ^{134}Cs and ^{137}Cs to the environment

(continued)

Table B2 (continued)

4	**Refer to look-up tables showing checklists of major constraints for each management option, including those for waste disposal**
	Table 6.6 provides information on the key constraints for each option There is only one option to be implemented before arrival of the plume (closing air intake systems at processing factories). For most foreseeable future NREs, some form of early notification of a possible release would be expected, making implementation more likely, especially at increasing distances from the site of the NRE Clean feeding is constrained by the availability of alternative clean feeds and suitable areas (either fenced areas or barns) in which to provide a supply of clean feed. It is early in the growing season, so there is unlikely to be any stored feed available. There are no barns in the affected upland areas and the erection of fences is not permitted as it is a national park. This option can be eliminated Live monitoring is constrained by the availability of NaI detectors and trained personnel, which would take time to organise. Live monitoring would therefore be a medium- to long-term option Select alternative land use and slaughtering of livestock (for disposal) is a radical option that should only be considered when all other options have been excluded. As there are alternatives, these options can be eliminated Selective grazing requires the availability of less contaminated pasture nearby. In this case, improved lowland pasture can be found in close proximity to the upland areas; it is already used by farmers to 'finish' the lambs over a 4-week period prior to the lambs being sent to market The administration of AFCF boli to ruminants and the distribution of AFCF salt licks in the upland areas require a supply of AFCF boli and AFCF salt licks, which would not be readily available and take time to manufacture. This would be a medium- to long-term option Restrictions on the entry of contaminated lamb into the food chain are based on statutory food restriction orders and will be legally binding, irrespective of any constraints. Where there is uncertainty that contaminated lamb products may have entered the food chain before restrictions had been put in place, product recall is a possible option In situations where unique traditional lifestyles need to be protected, a special case for raising intervention levels to above those dictated by statutory restrictions can be considered. This would only be appropriate in the absence of other management options, so it is unnecessary in this scenario Similarly, the salting of meat to reduce activity concentrations of ^{134}Cs and ^{137}Cs to below OILs can be considered when other options for reducing contamination in live animals are not possible. This is not necessary in this scenario Provided management options such as selective grazing and live monitoring are put in place, there should not be large volumes of sheep or lamb meat requiring disposal Burial of carcasses depends on the availability and suitability of land for the construction of a purpose-built burial pit Rendering and landfill depend on availability of facilities in the area and capacity of the landfill to take biodegradable material At this stage, the following management options still need to be considered:

Live animals: Change in husbandry	Animal products
Live monitoring	Close air intake at processing plant
Selective grazing	Product recall
Live animals: Use of additives	Restrict entry into food chain
Administer AFCF boli to ruminants	Disposal of meat
Distribution of AFCF salt licks	Burial
	Landfill
	Rendering

(continued)

Table B2 (continued)

5	**Refer to look-up table showing effectiveness of management options**
	Table 6.7 provides information on effectiveness. Selective grazing and the administration of AFCF boli are up to 80% effective. Live monitoring has the potential to be up 100% effective. In contrast, the effectiveness of AFCF salt licks is highly variable within a flock; they only work if animals are salt deficient. In this scenario, the affected area is close to the sea, so AFCF salt licks would not be effective and can be eliminated In terms of animal products, closing air intake at food processing plants, product recall and restricting entry into the food chain are all up to 100% effective
6	**Refer to look-up tables showing management options that incur an additional dose to those involved in their implementation either directly or through the management of any secondary wastes produced**
	Tables 6.8 and 6.9 provide information on doses and waste production from the implementation of management options Selective grazing involves the gathering and movement of livestock from the contaminated area to less contaminated pasture which incurs a small additional dose to the farmer Administration of AFCF boli and live monitoring may also incur a small additional dose to veterinary professionals or monitoring personnel, depending on where these activities take place None of these options produce waste Closing air intake systems at processing plants and the raising of intervention levels do not incur an additional dose or generate waste The placing of restrictions on the entry of sheep meat (lamb) into the food chain has the potential to generate waste if no other actions are taken; the management of this waste would lead to additional doses to those carrying out disposal All of the disposal options incur an additional dose to implementers. Burial and landfill also have the potential to expose members of the public to secondary wastes derived from these processes
7	**Refer to individual datasheets (Annex A) for all options remaining in the selection table, and note any further constraints**
	This step involves a detailed analysis of all remaining options by careful consideration of the relevant datasheets. It can only be done on a site-specific basis and in close consultation with local stakeholders to take into account local circumstances
8	**Based on Steps 1– 7, select and combine options that should be considered as part of the recovery strategy**
	Options for maintaining lamb production **Pre-deposition phase**: Close air intake systems at meat processing plants (requires adequate notification) **Urgent–early phase**: Restrict entry of contaminated lamb into food chain; and product recall where there is uncertainty that contaminated lamb products may have entered the food chain before restrictions had been put in place **Early–late phase**: Selective grazing by moving sheep from upland pasture to less contaminated lowland pasture. Where this is not possible, administer AFCF boli. Live monitoring of animals following selective grazing/administration of AFCF boli, to confirm activity concentration in meat < OIL, before sale *Options for disposing of waste* Provided selective grazing and AFCF boli can be implemented, the amount of waste generated will be small. Rendering of carcasses to reduce volume, followed by disposal to landfill. If landfill is unavailable, burial of carcasses in purpose-built pits should be considered

Table B3 Worked example to illustrate a strategy for iodine and caesium contamination of poultry (backyard production)

Radionuclides: ^{131}I, ^{134}Cs, ^{137}Cs
Product: Meat and eggs (chicken, turkey, etc.)
Time of year: End of growing season
Type of land: Poor quality pasture Southeastern Europe (backyard production)
Duration that OILs are exceeded: Weeks–months

Step	Action
1	**Identify one or more production systems that are likely to be/have been contaminated**
	It is meat production systems that have been affected. Management options are required for producing poultry meat with activity concentrations below the OILs. It is likely that these options will have to be in place for a period of several months, while activity concentrations of ^{134}Cs and ^{137}Cs decrease
2	**Refer to selection table for specific production systems**
	Table 6.2 provides a list of management options for all types of meat production (not just poultry), including those for waste disposal. Many of these options can be disregarded for backyard production systems: change in hunting season (for free-ranging, wild animals such as deer); live monitoring (ruminants only); selective grazing (ruminants only); addition of clay minerals to feed (ruminants only); administration of AFCF boli (ruminants only); distribution of salt licks (free-ranging ruminants); closing air intake systems at processing plants (intensive production); raising intervention levels (protected lifestyles such as Saami reindeer herders) Therefore, there are 6 options for live animals, 4 options for meat products and 5 options for disposal that still need to be considered:

Live animals: Change in husbandry	Meat products
Clean feeding	Provision of monitoring equipment
Manipulate slaughter times	Product recall
Select alternative land use	Restrict entry into food chain
Slaughtering (culling) of livestock	Salting of meat
Live animals: Use of additives	Disposal of meat
Addition of AFCF to feed	Burial of carcasses
Addition of calcium to feed	Burning of carcasses
	Incineration
	Landfill
	Rendering

Step	Action
3	**Refer to look-up tables showing applicability of management options, including those for waste disposal, for the radionuclide being considered**
	Tables 6.4 and 6.5 provide information on the applicability of options for ^{131}I, ^{134}Cs and ^{137}Cs If ^{131}I was the only radionuclide present in the environment, several additional management options could be eliminated, either because they are specific for caesium or strontium or because they are unsuitable for radionuclides with short physical half-lives. However, as ^{134}Cs and ^{137}Cs are also involved in contamination of meat in this scenario, only 3 options can be eliminated: addition of calcium to feed (strontium only); burning of carcasses; and incineration of carcasses (volatilisation of ^{131}I, ^{134}Cs, ^{137}Cs and release to the environment)

(continued)

Table B3 (continued)

<table>
<tr><td>4</td><td colspan="2">Refer to look-up tables showing checklists of major constraints for each management option, including those for waste disposal</td></tr>
<tr><td></td><td colspan="2">Table 6.6 provides information on the key constraints for each option
Clean feeding not only depends on the availability of alternative supplies of clean feed but also on suitable housing to prevent the animals going outside and ingesting contaminated feed, vegetation and soil. Manipulating slaughter times by prolonging slaughter may be possible if housing and clean feed is available. As the NRE occurred at the end of the growing season, it is likely that alternative clean feed would be available to support prolonging slaughter
The addition of AFCF to feed reduces the gut uptake of any caesium present in the diet. However, it is likely that AFCF will not be immediately available for incorporation into feed, so this should be considered as a later option
The selection of an alternative land use and slaughtering (culling) of poultry (for disposal) only need to be considered if there are no other viable options for reducing contamination in the live animals or meat products. This is unlikely to be situation in this scenario as both clean feeding, manipulation of slaughter times and addition of AFCF to feed are viable alternatives
Restrictions on the entry of contaminated poultry into the food chain are based on statutory food restriction orders and will be legally binding, irrespective of any constraints. Where there is uncertainty that contaminated poultry products may have entered the food chain before restrictions had been put in place, product recall is a possible option
Where poultry is for home consumption (by the farmer and his/her family), access to/ provision of monitoring equipment to measure radionuclide content in meat can be useful. However, it takes time to obtain monitoring kits and to train personnel, so this should be considered as a later option
The salting of meat can be considered for poultry with activity concentrations of ^{134}Cs and ^{137}Cs above OILs, either on a commercial basis or for home consumption. If carried out commercially, there is a risk of generating mistrust in the food chain. However, if food supplies are limited, this is a viable option
Burial of carcasses depends on the availability and suitability of land for the construction of a purpose-built burial pit
Rendering and landfill depend on availability of facilities in the area and capacity of the landfill to take biodegradable material
At this stage, the following management options still need to be considered:</td></tr>
<tr><td></td><td><u>Live animals: Change in husbandry</u></td><td><u>Meat products</u></td></tr>
<tr><td></td><td>Clean feeding</td><td>Provision of monitoring equipment</td></tr>
<tr><td></td><td>Manipulate slaughter times</td><td>Product recall</td></tr>
<tr><td></td><td></td><td>Restrict entry into food chain</td></tr>
<tr><td></td><td></td><td>Salting of meat</td></tr>
<tr><td></td><td><u>Live animals: Use of additives</u></td><td><u>Disposal of meat</u></td></tr>
<tr><td></td><td>Addition of AFCF to feed</td><td>Burial of carcasses</td></tr>
<tr><td></td><td></td><td>Landfill</td></tr>
<tr><td></td><td></td><td>Rendering</td></tr>
</table>

(continued)

Table B3 (continued)

5	**Refer to look-up table showing effectiveness of management options**
	Table 6.7 provides information on effectiveness. Clean feeding accompanied by the housing of poultry can be up to 100% effective for ^{131}I, ^{134}Cs and ^{137}Cs. The addition of AFCF to feed is also effective for ^{134}Cs and ^{137}Cs (~ 80%). In contrast, manipulation of slaughter time is not very effective, and with other more effective options available, this option can be eliminated In terms of animal products, provision of monitoring equipment, product recall and restricting entry into the food chain are all up to 100% effective for ^{131}I, ^{134}Cs and ^{137}Cs. The salting of meat can be up to 80% effective for ^{134}Cs and ^{137}Cs depending on size of portions treated and duration of treatment
6	**Refer to look-up tables showing management options that incur an additional dose to those involved in their implementation either directly or through the management of any secondary wastes produced**
	Tables 6.8 and 6.9 provide information on doses and waste production from the implementation of management options Clean feeding of housed poultry can incur very small incremental doses to the farmer from the handling of waste in the form of contaminated slurry that may be generated by housed animals during their period of clean feeding. This only happens if the animals were living outdoors after deposition of radionuclides from the NRE. The doses will be very low and not preclude implementation The addition of AFCF to feed does not result in any incremental doses to the farmer or the generation of any waste The placing of restrictions on the entry of poultry into the food chain as well as product recall generates waste, the management of which leads to additional doses to those carrying out disposal. A dose assessment will be required for the disposal routes selected The provision of monitoring equipment can incur a very small incremental dose to those going into a contaminated area to provide the service. The doses will be very low and not preclude implementation The salting of meat gives rise to a small additional dose to those handling the meat. The wastes from processing will be contaminated and the handling of these will incur additional doses. A dose assessment will be required for commercial facilities for the disposal routes selected All of the disposal options incur an additional dose to implementers. Burial and landfill also have the potential to expose members of the public to secondary wastes derived from these processes
7	**Refer to individual datasheets (Annex A) for all options remaining in the selection table, and note any further constraints**
	This step involves a detailed analysis of all remaining options by careful consideration of the relevant datasheets. It can only be done on a site-specific basis and in close consultation with local stakeholders to take into account local circumstances
8	**Based on Steps 1–7, select and combine options that should be considered as part of the recovery strategy**
	Options for producing clean meat/maintaining meat production **Pre-deposition phase**: There are no management options applicable **Urgent phase**: Restrict entry of contaminated poultry into food chain; and product recall where there is uncertainty that contaminated poultry may have entered the food chain before restrictions had been put in place **Early–late phase**: Provide housing and clean feed until levels of ^{131}I, ^{134}Cs and ^{137}Cs in backyard environment decrease; addition of AFCF to feed; provision of monitoring equipment particularly where poultry is for consumption by farmer and family; salting of meat where food supplies are limited ***Options for disposing of waste*** Rendering of carcasses to reduce volume, followed by disposal to landfill. If landfill is unavailable, burial of carcasses in purpose-built pits should be considered

Permissions

All chapters in this book were first published by Springer; hereby published with permission under the Creative Commons Attribution License or equivalent. Every chapter published in this book has been scrutinized by our experts. Their significance has been extensively debated. The topics covered herein carry significant information for a comprehensive understanding. They may even be implemented as practical applications or may be referred to as a beginning point for further studies.

The contributors of this book come from diverse backgrounds, making this book a truly international effort. We would like to thank all the contributing authors for lending their expertise to make the book truly unique. They have played a crucial role in the development of this book. Without their invaluable contributions this book wouldn't have been possible. They have made vital efforts to compile up to date information on the varied aspects of this subject to make this book a valuable addition to the collection of many professionals and students.

This book was conceptualized with the vision of imparting up-to-date and integrated information in this field. To ensure the same, a matchless editorial board was set up. Every individual on the board went through rigorous rounds of assessment to prove their worth. After which they invested a large part of their time researching and compiling the most relevant data for our readers.

The editorial board has been involved in producing this book since its inception. They have spent rigorous hours researching and exploring the diverse topics which have resulted in the successful publishing of this book. They have passed on their knowledge of decades through this book. To expedite this challenging task, the publisher supported the team at every step. A small team of assistant editors was also appointed to further simplify the editing procedure and attain best results for the readers.

Apart from the editorial board, the designing team has also invested a significant amount of their time in understanding the subject and creating the most relevant covers. They scrutinized every image to scout for the most suitable representation of the subject and create an appropriate cover for the book.

The publishing team has been an ardent support to the editorial, designing and production team. Their endless efforts to recruit the best for this project, has resulted in the accomplishment of this book. They are a veteran in the field of academics and their pool of knowledge is as vast as their experience in printing. Their expertise and guidance has proved useful at every step. Their uncompromising quality standards have made this book an exceptional effort. Their encouragement from time to time has been an inspiration for everyone.

The publisher and the editorial board hope that this book will prove to be a valuable piece of knowledge for students, practitioners and scholars across the globe.

Index

www.ingramcontent.com/pod-product-compliance
Lightning Source LLC
LaVergne TN
LVHW011513200926
848484LV00001B/34